IMPROVING HEALTH LITERACY WITHIN A STATE

WORKSHOP SUMMARY

Maria Hewitt, *Rapporteur*

Roundtable on Health Literacy

Board on Population Health and Public Health Practice

INSTITUTE OF MEDICINE
OF THE NATIONAL ACADEMIES

THE NATIONAL ACADEMIES PRESS
Washington, D.C.
www.nap.edu

THE NATIONAL ACADEMIES PRESS   500 Fifth Street, N.W.   Washington, DC 20001

NOTICE: The project that is the subject of this report was approved by the Governing Board of the National Research Council, whose members are drawn from the councils of the National Academy of Sciences, the National Academy of Engineering, and the Institute of Medicine.

This study was supported by contracts between the National Academy of Sciences and the Agency for Healthcare Research and Quality (HHSP233200900537P), Health Resources and Services Administration (HHSH25034004T), American College of Physicians Foundation, Association of Health Insurance Plans, the East Bay Community Foundation; GlaxoSmithKline, Johnson & Johnson, Kaiser Permanente, Merck and Co., Inc., and the Missouri Foundation for Health (09-0290-HL-09). Any opinions, findings, conclusions, or recommendations expressed in this publication are those of the author(s) and do not necessarily reflect the view of the organizations or agencies that provided support for this project.

International Standard Book Number-13:   978-0-309-21572-5
International Standard Book Number-10:   0-309-21572-2

Additional copies of this report are available from the National Academies Press, 500 Fifth Street, N.W., Lockbox 285, Washington, DC 20055; (800) 624-6242 or (202) 334-3313 (in the Washington metropolitan area); Internet, http://www.nap.edu. For more information about the Institute of Medicine, visit the IOM home page at: **www.iom.edu.**

Copyright 2011 by the National Academy of Sciences. All rights reserved.

Printed in the United States of America

The serpent has been a symbol of long life, healing, and knowledge among almost all cultures and religions since the beginning of recorded history. The serpent adopted as a logotype by the Institute of Medicine is a relief carving from ancient Greece, now held by the Staatliche Museen in Berlin.

Suggested citation: IOM (Institute of Medicine). 2011. *Improving Health Literacy Within a State: Workshop Summary*. Washington, DC: The National Academies Press.

*"Knowing is not enough; we must apply.
Willing is not enough; we must do."*
—Goethe

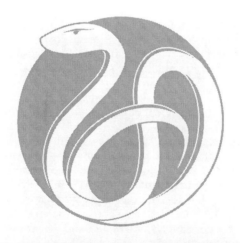

INSTITUTE OF MEDICINE
OF THE NATIONAL ACADEMIES

Advising the Nation. Improving Health.

THE NATIONAL ACADEMIES
Advisers to the Nation on Science, Engineering, and Medicine

The **National Academy of Sciences** is a private, nonprofit, self-perpetuating society of distinguished scholars engaged in scientific and engineering research, dedicated to the furtherance of science and technology and to their use for the general welfare. Upon the authority of the charter granted to it by the Congress in 1863, the Academy has a mandate that requires it to advise the federal government on scientific and technical matters. Dr. Ralph J. Cicerone is president of the National Academy of Sciences.

The **National Academy of Engineering** was established in 1964, under the charter of the National Academy of Sciences, as a parallel organization of outstanding engineers. It is autonomous in its administration and in the selection of its members, sharing with the National Academy of Sciences the responsibility for advising the federal government. The National Academy of Engineering also sponsors engineering programs aimed at meeting national needs, encourages education and research, and recognizes the superior achievements of engineers. Dr. Charles M. Vest is president of the National Academy of Engineering.

The **Institute of Medicine** was established in 1970 by the National Academy of Sciences to secure the services of eminent members of appropriate professions in the examination of policy matters pertaining to the health of the public. The Institute acts under the responsibility given to the National Academy of Sciences by its congressional charter to be an adviser to the federal government and, upon its own initiative, to identify issues of medical care, research, and education. Dr. Harvey V. Fineberg is president of the Institute of Medicine.

The **National Research Council** was organized by the National Academy of Sciences in 1916 to associate the broad community of science and technology with the Academy's purposes of furthering knowledge and advising the federal government. Functioning in accordance with general policies determined by the Academy, the Council has become the principal operating agency of both the National Academy of Sciences and the National Academy of Engineering in providing services to the government, the public, and the scientific and engineering communities. The Council is administered jointly by both Academies and the Institute of Medicine. Dr. Ralph J. Cicerone and Dr. Charles M. Vest are chair and vice chair, respectively, of the National Research Council.

www.national-academies.org

PLANNING COMMITTEE ON UNDERSTANDING WHAT WORKS IN HEALTH LITERACY ACROSS A STATE[1]

SHARON BARRETTT, Health Literacy Staff Consultant, Association of Clinicians for the Underserved
CAROLYN COCOTAS, Senior Vice President, Quality and Corporate Compliance, F.E.G.S. Health and Human Services
JEAN KRAUSE, Executive Vice President and CEO, American College of Physicians Foundation
RUTH PARKER, Professor of Medicine, Emory University School of Medicine
DEAN SCHILLINGER, Professor of Medicine in Residence, University of California San Francisco

---

[1] Institute of Medicine planning committees are solely responsible for organizing the workshop, identifying topics, and choosing speakers. The responsibility for the published workshop summary rests with the workshop rapporteur and the institution.

ROUNDTABLE ON HEALTH LITERACY[1]

GEORGE ISHAM (*Chair*), Medical Director and Chief Health Officer, HealthPartners
SHARON E. BARRETT, Health Literacy Staff Consultant, Association of Clinicians for the Underserved
CINDY BRACH, Senior Health Policy Researcher, Center for Delivery, Organization, and Markets, Agency for Healthcare Research and Quality
CAROLYN COCOTAS, Senior Vice President, Quality and Corporate Compliance, F.E.G.S. Health and Human Services System
ARTHUR CULBERT, President and CEO, Health Literacy Missouri
MICHAEL L. DAVIS, Senior Vice President, Human Resources, General Mills, Inc.
BENARD P. DREYER, Professor of Pediatrics, New York University School of Medicine, and Chair, American Academy of Pediatrics Health Literacy Program Advisory Committee
LEONARD EPSTEIN, Senior Advisor, Clinical Quality and Culture, Health Resources and Services
DEBBIE FRITZ, Director, Policy and Standards, Health Management Innovations Division, GlaxoSmithKline
MARTHA GRAGG, Vice President of Program, Missouri Foundation for Health
LINDA HARRIS, Team Leader, Health Communication and eHealth Team, Office of Disease Prevention and Health Promotion, U.S. Department of Health and Human Services
BETSY L. HUMPHREYS, Deputy Director, National Library of Medicine, National Institutes of Health
JEAN KRAUSE, Executive Vice President and CEO, American College of Physicians Foundation
MARGARET LOVELAND, Global Medical Affairs, Merck & Co., Inc.
PATRICK McGARRY, Assistant Division Director, Scientific Activities Division, American Academy of Family Physicians
RUTH PARKER, Professor of Medicine, Emory University School of Medicine
YOLANDA PARTIDA, Director, National Program Office, Hablamos Juntos, University of California, San Francisco, Fresno Center for Medical Education & Research

---

[1] Institute of Medicine forums and roundtables do not issue, review, or approve individual documents. The responsibility for the published workshop summary rests with the workshop rapporteur and the institution.

CLARENCE PEARSON, Consultant, Globabl Health Leadership and Management
SUSAN PISANO, Director of Communications, America's Health Insurance Plans
ANDREW PLEASANT, Health Literacy and Research Director, Canyon Ranch Institute
SCOTT C. RATZAN, Vice President, Global Health, Johnson & Johnson
WILL ROSS, Associate Dean for Diversity, Associate Professor of Medicine, Washington University School of Medicine
PAUL M. SCHYVE, Senior Vice President, The Joint Commission
PATRICK WAYTE, Vice President, Marketing and Health Education, American Heart Association
WINSTON F. WONG, Medical Director, Community Benefit, Disparities Improvement and Quality Initiatives, Kaiser Permanente

Study Staff

LYLA M. HERNANDEZ, Staff Director
CHINA DICKERSON, Senior Project Assistant (until December 2, 2010)
ANGELA MARTIN, Senior Project Assistant (beginning November 1, 2010)
ROSE MARIE MARTINEZ, Director, Board on Population Health and Public Health Practice

Reviewers

This report has been reviewed in draft form by individuals chosen for their diverse perspectives and technical expertise, in accordance with procedures approved by the National Research Council's Report Review Committee. The purpose of this independent review is to provide candid and critical comments that will assist the institution in making its published report as sound as possible and to ensure that the report meets institutional standards for objectivity, evidence, and responsiveness to the study charge. The review comments and draft manuscript remain confidential to protect the integrity of the process. We wish to thank the following individuals for their review of this report:

Martha Gragg, Medical University of South Carolina
John Gutierrez, University of California Los Angeles School of Dentistry
Lauren McCormack, RTI International
Antronette Yancy, University of California Los Angeles Kaiser Permanente Center for Health Equity

Although the reviewers listed above have provided many constructive comments and suggestions, they did not endorse the final draft of the report before its release. The review of this report was overseen by **Harold J. Fallon,** Medical University of South Carolina. Appointed by the Institute of Medicine, he was responsible for making certain that an independent examination of this report was carried out in accordance with institutional procedures and that all review comments were carefully considered. Responsibility for the final content of this report rests entirely with the rapporteur and the institution.

Acknowledgments

The sponsors of the Institute of Medicine Roundtable on Health Literacy made it possible to plan and conduct the workshop, Understanding What Works in Improving Health Literacy Within a State. Sponsors from the U.S. Department of Health and Human Services are the Agency for Healthcare Research and Quality and the Health Resources and Services Administration. Non-federal sponsorship was provided by the American College of Physicians Foundation; the Association of Health Insurance Plans; the East Bay Community Foundation; GlaxoSmithKline; Johnson & Johnson; Kaiser Permanente; Merck and Co., Inc.; and the Missouri Foundation for Health.

The Roundtable wishes to express its gratitude to the following speakers for their thoughtful and stimulating presentations: Mary Ann Abrams, Ellen Beck, Arthur Culbert, Terry Davis, Ariella Herman, Carol Mangione, Alfred E. Osborne, Jr., Rima Rudd, Dean Schillinger, Pam C. Silberman, Cynthia Solomon, and Eugene Washington. The Roundtable also wishes to express its appreciation to the planning committee for their hard work in putting together an excellent workshop agenda. Members of the planning committee are Sharon Barrett, Carolyn Cocotas, Jean Krause, Ruth Parker, and Dean Schillinger.

Contents

1 INTRODUCTION   1

2 KEYNOTE ADDRESS   3
   Opening Remarks and Introduction of Keynote Speaker, 3
   Overview of the Role of the University in Improving Health
      Literacy Statewide, 4

3 STATE-BASED MODELS TO IMPROVE HEALTH LITERACY   7
   The Road to Regional Transformation: The North
      Carolina Experience, 7
   The Iowa Experience: Creating a Shared Vision for Health
      Literacy in Iowa, 12
   Discussion, 17
   The Missouri Experience, 21
   Louisiana Statewide Health Literacy Initiative, 24
   Discussion, 29

4 THE ROLE OF THE UNIVERSITY IN IMPROVING STATES'
   HEALTH LITERACY   33
   How the University Can Advance State Health Literacy, 33
   Workforce Training and Preparedness, 42
   Discussion, 48

5	IMPROVING HEALTH LITERACY AT THE COMMUNITY LEVEL	51

New York City Mayor's Initiative on Health Literacy, 51
MiVIA, 56
Empowering Parents, Benefiting Children, Creating Strong Foundations for Health: Improving Health Literacy Through the Head Start Program, 59
Health Literacy at the University of California, San Diego, Student-Run Free Clinic Project and Fellowship in Underserved Health Care: Learnings, 65
Discussion, 71

6	CLOSING REMARKS	75
	REFERENCES	79

APPENDIXES

A	ACRONYMS	83
B	WORKSHOP AGENDA	85
C	WORKSHOP SPEAKER BIOSKETCHES	89

Tables, Figures, and Boxes

TABLES

2-1 Experience of Collaboration in Decision Making, Simulated Model, 5
2-2 Groups Involved in Health Literacy: Definitions, 6

4-1 Results of Informal Survey of University of California Health Professional Schools' Health Literacy Curriculum, 45

5-1 Parents' Sources of Help When a Child Is Sick, 63
5-2 Outcomes of 182 Diabetic Patients Seen at the UCSD Free Clinic and Assessed at 1 Year, 68

FIGURES

5-1 HCI health improvement project, 61
5-2 HCI strategic implementation, 61
5-3 Overview of the Head Start intervention, 64

BOXES

3-1 Iowa Health Literacy Sponsors and Their Projects, 13
3-2 Iowa Health Literacy Steering Work Group Membership, 14
3-3 Principles of Health Literacy Iowa, 14

4-1 Study Objectives, 37
4-2 Anticipated Study Outcomes, 37

5-1 Guidebook Outline, 55
5-2 Goals of the HCI Health Literacy Program, 60

1

Introduction

Health literacy is the degree to which individuals can obtain, process, and understand the basic health information and services they need to make appropriate health decisions. Nearly half of all American adults—90 million people—have inadequate health literacy to navigate the healthcare system (IOM, 2004).

The Institute of Medicine (IOM) convened the Roundtable on Health Literacy to address issues raised in the report, *Health Literacy: A Prescription to End Confusion* (IOM, 2004). The roundtable brings together leaders from the federal government, foundations, health plans, associations, and private companies to discuss challenges facing health literacy practice and research and to identify approaches to promote health literacy in both the public and private sectors. The roundtable also serves to educate the public, press, and policy makers regarding issues related to health literacy. The roundtable sponsors workshops for members and the public to discuss approaches to resolve key challenges.

An area of interest for the roundtable is ways in which various organizations and individuals within a state can work to improve health literacy within that state. As a result, the roundtable cosponsored a workshop with the University of California, Los Angeles (UCLA), Anderson School of Management in Los Angeles on November 30, 2010. The workshop focused on understanding what works to improve health literacy across a state, including how various stakeholders have a role in improving health literacy. The focus of the workshop was on presentations and discussions that address (1) the clinical impacts of health literacy improvement approaches; (2) economic outcomes of health literacy implementation; and (3) how various stakeholders can affect health literacy.

The workshop was organized by an independent planning committee in accordance with the procedures of the National Academy of Sciences. The planning group included Sharon Barrett, Darren DeWalt, Jean Krause, Ruth Parker, Dean Schillinger, and Carol Teutsch. The role of the workshop planning committee was limited to planning the workshop. Planning committee members developed the agenda topics, and selected and invited expert speakers and discussants to address identified topics. Unlike a consensus committee report, a workshop summary may not contain conclusions and recommendations. Therefore, this summary has been prepared by the workshop rapporteur as a factual summary of what occurred at the workshop. All views presented in the report are those of workshop participants. The report does not contain any findings or recommendations by the planning committee or the roundtable.

The workshop was moderated by roundtable chair, George Isham, and featured presentations and discussion. Chapter 2 presents a summary of the keynote address on the role of the university in improving health literacy. Chapter 3 focuses on state-based models to improve health literacy. In Chapter 4, the role of the university in improving health literacy statewide is explored further. Chapter 5 covers improving health literacy at the community level. Chapter 6 follows with a general discussion of the day's proceedings.

2

Keynote Address

OPENING REMARKS AND INTRODUCTION OF KEYNOTE SPEAKER

Alfred E. Osborne, Jr., Ph.D., M.B.A., M.A.
Anderson School of Management

Osborne emphasized the importance of health literacy and noted that the U.S. Department of Health and Human Services (HHS) has made improving the nation's health literacy a national priority. In his view, having the Anderson School of Management cosponsor a workshop on health literacy with the Institute of Medicine (IOM) is consistent with the school's mission of enhancing the administrative skills of leaders within organizations that are addressing the needs of underserved communities. For example, the school's Health Care Institute (HCI) has experience training Head Start Program leadership, staff, and participants. HCI also has a relationship with the Health Resources and Services Administration (HRSA) in its work with community health centers. Osborne welcomed roundtable members, speakers, and the audience to the UCLA campus and introduced the keynote speaker, A. Eugene Washington.

OVERVIEW OF THE ROLE OF THE UNIVERSITY IN IMPROVING HEALTH LITERACY STATEWIDE

A. Eugene Washington, M.D., M.Sc.
UCLA Health Sciences and
David Geffen School of Medicine at UCLA

Washington addressed four questions pertaining to health literacy in his presentation: Why is health literacy important? Who must understand its importance? How can its importance best be conveyed? What is the role of the academic community in addressing the needs of health literacy? Washington pointed out that the focus of the workshop is state-based approaches to health literacy, but he emphasized the global nature of the problem of low health literacy. He suggested that what is learned from local and statewide efforts could be translated to affect care around the world.

The transitive property states that, "If a = b and b = c, then a = c." This formula is used in philosophy, especially in the understanding of logic. Using the transitive property in the context of health literacy and quality health care means that if the quality of health care (a) depends on effective patient provider communication (b) and effective provider communication depends on understanding the health literacy level of the patient (c), then the quality of care depends on understanding the patient's health literacy level. In short, the quality of care depends on both the patient's level of literacy and the effectiveness of provider communication. This transitive property can also be applied in the context of population health. The ability to improve the overall health status of a population or a community depends on the effectiveness of communication with the entire community. And that, in turn, depends on understanding the health literacy level of the population.

The IOM report, *Crossing the Quality Chasm*, stated that health care should be safe, effective, patient centered, timely, efficient, and equitable (IOM, 2001). If care is patient centered, individuals leave their clinical encounter with the understanding that their specific needs have been met. Timely care means that necessary interventions are available and the processes of care are efficient. Washington observed that poor communication is often what leads to medication errors. A clinician may choose the wrong therapy for a patient because he or she did not understand what the patient was saying. Alternatively, a patient may not take medications appropriately because the clinician did not give specific instructions.

In early research that examined the elements of patient-provider communication and shared decision making, episodes of care were videotaped with the provider knowing that the encounter was being recorded. Patients and providers rated the encounters in terms of whether "part-

TABLE 2-1 Experience of Collaboration in Decision Making, Simulated Model

Shared Decision Making	Positive	Negative
Present	True partnering 22%	False partnering 38%
Absent	Assumed partnering 21%	Unwilling partnering 19%

SOURCE: Adapted from Saba et al., 2006.

nering" in care occurred. True shared decision making occurred only 22 percent of the time while simulated shared decision making occurred 38 percent of the time (Table 2-1).

When thinking about improving health literacy, Washington said, it is important to understand the perspectives of the various parties that listen to health literacy messages. The reaction to the message will depend on the role in which the recipient views him or herself. Yet the deliverer of the message often views the recipients as uniform. Various roles of the recipient are those of audience, customer, constituent, partner, and stakeholder (Table 2-2).

Those that need to be engaged to effectively understand and communicate the importance of health literacy include patients, providers, employers, payers, policy makers, communities and populations, community leaders, researchers, educators, and communicators and disseminators. When developing messages it is important to distinguish who is the primary audience, customer, constituent, partner, or stakeholder. It may also be necessary to think about whether particular groups are the primary, secondary, or tertiary audience.

There is value in partnering with the communications industry because of its great expertise in using media to communicate effectively, Washington said. This key group, which has not been given sufficient attention, should be viewed as a principal partner and a major stakeholder in both education and research efforts. Members of this group can also be involved in efforts to intervene and improve health status.

In terms of the academic community, health sciences centers, schools of education, and schools of communication have a major role to play in conveying the importance of health literacy and furthering health literacy practice. The academic community more broadly has a key role to play in teaching and expanding the relevant workforce and in advancing research methods and knowledge of what works.

Projections of health professional shortages in California made by HRSA can provide opportunities insofar as they represent positions for

TABLE 2-2 Groups Involved in Health Literacy: Definitions

Audience	The group of spectators at a public event; listeners or viewers collectively, as in attendance at a theater or concert. A regular public that manifests interest, support, enthusiasm, or the like; a following
Constituent	A person who authorizes another to act on his or her behalf, as a voter in a district represented by an elected official
Customer	A person who purchases goods or services from another; buyer; patron
Partner	A person who shares or is associated with another in some action or endeavor; sharer; associate. A player on the same side or team as another
Stakeholder	A person or group not owning shares in an enterprise, but affected by, or having an interest in its operations, such as the employees, customers, and local community

SOURCE: Dictionary.com.

which individuals will have to be trained. Newly trained health personnel should be educated to understand the importance of health literacy and provide care that is linguistically appropriate, Washington said.

Educational institutions have played an important role in furthering the use of multidisciplinary, community-based, participatory research. Such research should include schools of business, engineering, education, and communication, along with the traditional disciplines in health sciences. Another area for involvement of the academic community relates to interventions to improve health literacy. Researchers in academic institutions are furthering the science of establishing what interventions are most effective. Interventions include communication strategies both at the individual level, and for populations at large. The development of methods, measurements, and standards are critical to understanding what works and to determine whether or not providers, institutions, organizations, and communities are providing care and messages that are at the appropriate health literacy level.

The educational enterprise must embrace the idea of a continuum of lifelong learning, not only for individuals and patients, but also for healthcare providers. Such an approach is needed in order to fully appreciate the dimensions of low health literacy and the opportunities to intervene and ensure high-quality health care. Low health literacy is not simply a local, state, or even a national problem. It is a global problem. The outcomes of forums such as the IOM workshop have broad implications with the potential for improving health worldwide, he concluded.

3

State-Based Models to Improve Health Literacy

THE ROAD TO REGIONAL TRANSFORMATION: THE NORTH CAROLINA EXPERIENCE

Pam C. Silberman, J.D., Dr.P.H.
North Carolina Institute of Medicine

The North Carolina Institute of Medicine (NCIOM) is a quasi-state agency chartered in 1983 by the State's General Assembly to

- study important health issues facing the state;
- provide nonpartisan advise to the North Carolina (NC) General Assembly and executive agencies to help improve health policies; and
- provide advice to health professionals, insurers, business leaders, and the public to improve the health of NC residents.

In 2007, the North Carolina Division of Public Health asked NCIOM to convene a task force to study health literacy in the state. In response, the Task Force on Health Literacy[1] was formed to bring together key health literacy stakeholders and partners from throughout the state to review research about health literacy challenges and identify potential solutions.

---

[1] The task force was supported through a grant from the Centers for Disease Control and Prevention (CDC).

The Task Force members, 50 in all, represented the broad spectrum of stakeholders in health including health care provider groups and associations, state and local health and education agencies, insurers, consumers, and adult literacy experts. In terms of state agency involvement, the task force included members representing the NC Division of Public Health, the NC Department of Health and Human Services (NC DHHS) Medicaid unit, and the state's Area Health Education Center (AHEC) program. A consensus driven process led to the formulation of 14 recommendations.

In formulating their 14 recommendations, the task force took a universal precaution approach which is one of ensuring that communications are clear for everyone, regardless of literacy level. The recommendations focused on improving health care communications for all populations within the state rather than attempting to improve the literacy level of the general public. A 2010 assessment of progress on implementing the task force recommendations found that progress had been made on 11 of the 14 recommendations. No action had been taken to implement the remaining 3 recommendations. Silberman pointed out that by bringing together the right partners, the Task Force's recommendations were generally implemented without the NCIOM's active involvement. The NCIOM is not an advocacy organization so this level of engagement was critical to the success of the initiative, she said.

One recommendation of the task force was to create a NC Health Literacy Center of Excellence charged with

- educating health professionals,
- identifying evidence-based guidelines or best practices for health communications,
- disseminating health education materials, and
- assisting adult literacy professionals.

While a new center was not created, many of the recommended functions of the proposed center are now being carried out by the North Carolina (NC) Program on Health Literacy (http://www.nchealthliteracy.org/) and the NC Health Literacy Council (http://www.uncg.edu/csr/healthliteracy/). The NC Program on Health Literacy is housed at the University of North Carolina at Chapel Hill. It is a research- and teaching-oriented program that is actively involved in the identification of best practices. With Agency for Healthcare Research and Quality (AHRQ) support, the program developed the Health Literacy Universal Precaution Toolkit that supports primary care practices. The toolkit can be accessed at http://www.ahrq.gov/qual/literacy/.

The NC Health Literacy Council is housed at the University of North Carolina at Greensboro. The council primarily works with adult literacy and health literacy groups and has created local health literacy councils in several counties. The council also works with health care providers. Checklists are used to see whether providers and academic health centers are using clear communications and effective health literacy tools.

Another task force recommendation was to provide more education on health literacy to health professionals. Older providers who were educated many years ago often do not know about or understand the concept of health literacy, Silberman said. Reaching out to providers who have been in practice for a while is a challenge. While progress in improving health professional understanding of health literacy has been made, much remains to be accomplished. For example, during a 2008 meeting with about 50 physicians in Fayetteville, NC, none had ever heard of the term *health literacy*. In contrast, all of the students at the School of Public Health have heard this term. Several approaches are being taken to improve in this area including the following:

- The community college system includes information on health literacy in all nursing courses addressing patient education.
- Individual didactic sessions are offered in medical schools, pharmacy programs, and public health schools.
- The Area Health Education Center (AHEC) program offers health literacy content in continuing education programs that are offered to health professionals.

There are significant challenges to reaching out to providers who have been in practice for some time. When the AHEC program initially offered health literacy workshops, there was little interest. However, when health literacy concepts were embedded into their other workshops around patient safety and patient communication, there was considerable interest. Health literacy is also embedded in the community college training for nurses.

In response to the problem of pharmacy errors and the general lack of understanding by consumers about how to take medication, the task force recommended that pharmacists provide medication counseling and that North Carolina foundations test new models to enhance the role of pharmacists as medication counselors. Subsequently, the NC Health and Wellness Trust fund created "ChecKmeds," a pharmacy counseling service available at no cost to seniors across the state. Other foundations are helping to fund dissemination activities.

Another recommendation of the task force called for the NC DHHS to review all consumer education materials for appropriate health literacy. The NC DHHS website materials must now be written at no greater than a 7th-grade reading level. In addition, specific materials targeted to the Medicaid population have been evaluated and tested for health literacy.

Prior to the work of the task force, each local Medicaid network was creating its own materials, which were never tested for health literacy. Educational materials targeted to people with chronic illnesses have all been reviewed by health literacy expert Darren DeWalt and his colleagues at the University of North Carolina. Approved materials are being used across the state. A library of patient management tools has also been created.

The task force also recommended that people within NC DHHS at both the state and local level be trained in health literacy so that they could more effectively communicate with community groups and consumers. Silberman reported that some divisions have implemented training programs and those that have accomplished the most include the following:

- The Division of Public Health, Children and Youth Branch, which requires training for state and local staff on health literacy.
- The Division of Mental Health, Developmental Disabilities, and Substance Abuse Services has two trained staff persons who work on literacy and cultural competency issues and disseminate materials to local agencies.
- The Medicaid program has a patient education workgroup with representatives from across the state.

Another task force recommendation addressed the need for foundations and insurers to fund efforts to use lay health advisors, group education sessions, and care managers to enhance patient education. Progress in this area includes

- the use of care managers and group medical visits within the Medicaid program;
- the use of community health workers within the Division of Public Health;
- the use of community health workers (including those serving the Hispanic community) and care managers at community health centers; and
- the implementation of a congregational nurse program to provide health education, including health literacy, to faith communities.

The task force also recommended that malpractice carriers incorporate health literacy education into risk management training. Medical Mutual Group, the state's largest physician malpractice carrier, has incorporated information about health literacy in their risk management training, and it has created a health literacy toolkit. The training emphasizes the importance of clear communication in minimizing malpractice risk.

Another Task Force recommendation was that health literacy initiatives should be implemented in English as a Second Language (ESL) programs, adult basic education, and adult literacy courses. A health-related curriculum called *Expecting the Best*, developed prior to the formation of the NCIOM Task Force, has been used to meet the needs of people with limited English proficiency in the community college system. Many community-based literacy organizations have also incorporated this curriculum and health literacy content into their programs.

There are, however, three areas where little progress has been made, Silverman said. First, the task force recommended that the NC Board of Pharmacy require improvements in prescription bottle labeling, but no progress has been made in this area. Second, the task force recommended tying insurance reimbursement to a requirement that health professionals receive health literacy training. Again, no progress has been made in this area; however, Silberman said that there is potential for progress as value-based purchasing and pay-for-performance reimbursement are considered and adopted. Finally, the Task Force recommended that a broad-based social marketing campaign be launched to encourage consumers to be more active in asking questions of their providers. A state-based social marketing campaign was not funded through the NC general assembly; however, AHRQ's health literacy campaign has been promoted nationally and is airing health literacy commercials on television.

The North Carolina program is continuing to conduct research, educate health providers and administrators, and develop health literacy materials and interventions. The NC Health Literacy Council continues their grassroots efforts to build community coalitions and improve health literacy throughout the state. The council had its first annual health literacy conference in late 2010 with more than 100 attendees. The professional education and training programs described earlier through AHEC, the Medical Mutual Group, and the academic health centers have continued. The NCIOM is now focused on how best to implement health reform in the state rather than being directly involved in health literacy. However, health literacy is embedded in other work of the institute.

Silberman concluded by pointing out that there are several components of health care reform that provide opportunities to incorporate health literacy into implementation plans. These include

- developing comparative insurance information for the health benefit exchange ("plain language") (Sec. 1311(e)(3)(B));
- considering new models of care to more fully engage consumers in self-management of chronic diseases and primary prevention; and
- using patient education materials (e.g., decision aids, research findings) (Secs. 3501, 3506, 3507).

Other provisions in the Patient Protection and Affordable Care Act related to health professional training, expanding the role of patient navigators, and working with underserved populations also provide opportunities to focus on health literacy. In addition to the NCIOM 2007 report and its update in 2010, the NCIOM published an entire *North Carolina Medical Journal* on patient-provider communication (NCIOM, 2007).

THE IOWA EXPERIENCE: CREATING A SHARED VISION FOR HEALTH LITERACY IN IOWA

Mary Ann Abrams, M.D., M.P.H.
Iowa Health System

Abrams, a pediatrician, used developmental terms to describe the status of Iowa's health literacy initiatives. If the state were a child, she said, it would be at the "preschool age" in terms of health literacy. It is walking around and learning, but it is still in need of support. And as has any preschooler, the state has exciting ideas and wonderful opportunities in its future.

Iowa began to develop health literacy initiatives with support from the Wellmark Foundation, the philanthropic arm of the state Blue Cross insurer. The foundation had health literacy as one of its priority funding areas. This focus was a result of the Institute of Medicine's identification of health literacy as necessary to achieving quality and transforming health care in the United States (IOM, 2004).

An informal survey of state activities in health literacy shows numerous efforts under way Several of the sponsors and their projects are listed in Box 3-1. The next step in developing statewide capacity for health literacy is to coordinate and strengthen these various activities.

The Iowa Health System, Iowa's largest integrated health system, initiated the Health Literacy Collaborative project in 2003 to improve health care quality and safety by fostering effective communication and enabling all patients to read, understand, and act upon health information. Health literacy teams have been established in collaborative settings, including 11 senior hospital affiliates, 15 rural hospitals, 140 clinics, and home health settings. The *Plan, Do, Study, Act* (PDSA)[2] model for improvement is used. The education and training provided to the teams succeeded in turning the project into a passion, Abrams said, and also persuaded leadership to

---

[2]"The Deming cycle or PDSA cycle is a continuous quality improvement model consisting of a logical sequence of four repetitive steps for continuous improvement and learning: Plan, Do, Study (Check), and Act." See http://www.valuebasedmanagement.net/methods_demingcycle.html (accessed August 25, 2011).

> **BOX 3-1**
> **Iowa Health Literacy Sponsors and Their Projects**
>
> | Sponsor | Project |
> |---|---|
> | • Iowa Health System | • Health Literacy Collaborative |
> | • Drake College of Pharmacy | • *Ask Me 3* research |
> | • Iowa Healthcare Collaborative | • Health Literacy Toolkit |
> | • New Readers of Iowa | • Adult Learner Conferences |
> | • University of Northern Iowa | • Iowa Center for Health Disparities |
> | • Iowa Chapter, American Academy of Pediatrics | • *Reach Out and Read Iowa* |
> | • University of Iowa Geriatric Education Center | • Health Literacy Faculty Training |
>
> SOURCE: Abrams, 2010.

champion the efforts. Instrumental to the project's success were involvement of adult learners and patients in the project's development, using multi-faceted approaches, and collaborating with interested partners.

Creating a shared vision for health literacy in Iowa began in October 2008 with a strategic planning day attended by over a hundred individuals from 40 to 50 different agencies and organizations. Nicole Lurie was invited as part of a 2-day visiting professorship.[3] Attendees were very enthusiastic and supportive of moving forward with health literacy initiatives. A white paper published following the meeting was widely circulated. From May 2009 to December 2010, a relatively large steering work group discussed the potential mission, functions, and infrastructure of a health literacy center, and how to launch and sustain such a center (Box 3-2).

The steering group agreed on a set of principles to guide health literacy efforts in Iowa (Box 3-3). These included the idea that a *universal* approach to health literacy would be taken. That approach recognizes that anyone can experience low health literacy, depending on the circumstances. Interventions, therefore, should be targeted to everyone, not only those who struggle with reading, and additional support should be available when needed. Another principle is to address both individual clinical encounters and, more broadly, populations at large. Collaborative part-

---

[3] Dr. Lurie, a prominent investigator in the area of health literacy, had been involved in the development of an interactive mapping tool to target low health literacy. She currently serves as the U.S. Department of Health and Human Services Deputy Assistant Secretary for Preparedness and Response.

> **BOX 3-2**
> **Iowa Health Literacy Steering Work Group Membership**
>
> Des Moines University
> DeskActive
> Governor's office
> Iowa Department of Education
> Iowa Department of Public Health
> Iowa Health System
> Iowa Healthcare Collaborative
> Iowa Hospital Association
> Iowa Medical Society
> Iowa Nurses Association
> Iowa Pharmacy Association
> Mercy Clinics, Inc.
> Nebraska Primary Care Association (community health centers)
> New Readers of Iowa
> Principal Financial Group
> University of Iowa
> - Center for Disabilities and Development
> - Geriatric Education Center
> University of Northern Iowa Centers on Iowa/Health Disparities and Immigration Leadership
> Wellmark Foundation
>
> SOURCE: Abrams, 2010.

> **BOX 3-3**
> **Principles of Health Literacy Iowa**
>
> - Universal issue
> - All aspects of health—individual and population-based
> - Cross-cutting
> - Fundamental to
>   o quality
>   o health reform
>   o reducing costs
> - Patient, family, adult learner involvement
> - Collaborative partnerships
> - Results-oriented sustained improvement
> - Response to National Plan to Improve Health Literacy
>
> SOURCE: Abrams, 2010.

nerships and the involvement of patients, families, and adult learners to achieve results, translate research into action, and sustain momentum are critical. The steering group's work has provided a platform to articulate Iowa's response to the U.S. Department of Health and Human Services National Action Plan to Improve Health Literacy (HHS, 2010).

The formal mission of Health Literacy Iowa (HLI) is to promote and facilitate the ability of all Iowans to use effective communication to optimize their health. The functions of HLI are to

- make the policy and business case for health literacy, raise awareness, and advocate for change;
- assist health care providers and organizations in using health literacy-related interventions and creating system change;
- educate and train;
- empower patients, families, and consumers;
- share resources;
- participate in research; and
- collaborate with state and regional partners.

HLI activities have taken place in three phases. Phase 1 occurred from July 2009 to December 2010 and included several informal initiatives. First, an Iowa-specific economic analysis was commissioned to provide economic data to make the business case for planned initiatives. As part of an awareness and branding initiative, a one-page description of the program was completed, a website was built, an electronic newsletter was circulated, and a number of presentations were delivered. This outreach led to the involvement of additional partners and the formation of a business development committee. Also during phase 1 adult learners and the New Readers of Iowa conducted a formal review of various materials and documents. That review was very informative and efforts are under way to develop and formalize this process so other materials can be reviewed and revised.

Faculty training and online learning modules were developed in collaboration with the Iowa Geriatric Education Center. Grant development activities included the development of reader friendly documents through an ADAPT[4] grant in partnership with the College of Pharmacy at the University of Iowa, and pursuit of a funding opportunity through the National Library of Medicine to support community libraries to function as the local "storefront" for HLI. The public library can provide access to health information using local librarians who are already information specialists. Finally, a steering work group partner was able to get an appropriation for HLI included within the federal appropriation request.

Phase 2 is the transition to an independent entity and will take place from January through December 2011. During this time HLI may be established as an independent not-for-profit organization. In the near term,

---

[4] ADAPT is the acronym for Adaptation and Dissemination of AHRQ (Agency for Healthcare Research and Quality) Comparative Effectiveness Research Products.

its goals will be to build capacity, develop clients and services, increase collaborative opportunities, and develop regional partnerships. The long-term goal is to establish HLI as the hub and the "go-to" place for health literacy information, resources, and connections.

HLI is considering a prototype regional health literacy cooperative with Minnesota, Wisconsin, Missouri, and other states. This cooperative would address capacity-building issues, and draw upon the expertise, skills, and strengths of each member state. HLI also intends to develop an extensive menu of education and training opportunities for a variety of audiences, including healthcare providers, employers, payers, and state agencies and to make material accessible using "plain language."[5]

HLI also intends to formalize the network of adult learners to support health literacy education, training, and services. This group is engaged and brings great value to the work of the organization. Other efforts will focus on developing the concept of library-based, community health literacy resource centers and Iowa-specific health literacy training materials, especially health literacy stories and videos. Finally, HLI intends to develop an evaluation and research agenda within Iowa and regionally.

Phase 3 of Health Literacy Iowa, the future endeavors, will take place in 2012 and beyond. These include advocating for health literacy by making the business and policy case for its role in transforming the healthcare system; articulating and integrating health literacy into health promotion, disease prevention, and disease management efforts; and augmenting programs in the Department of Education, especially those that integrate health literacy into early child development programs, and kindergarten through grade 12. HLI also intends to collaborate with educators at multiple levels including adult literacy and English as a Second Language (ESL). HLI expects to expand prevention strategies targeted to those at risk for low health literacy. Another important endeavor is to provide training, including technical assistance, consulting, and coaching. Priority areas for these activities include condition-specific initiatives, cultural and linguistic training, and interpretation services.

At the community or population level, HLI will focus on providing accessible materials and disseminating information to the public, employers, state agencies, legislators, and special groups (e.g., children). It will increase involvement in research and also continue its role as a convener and developer of partnerships at the state, regional, and national levels.

Abrams concluded her remarks by discussing lessons learned. She described HLI as a learning organization that continues to adapt and be flexible. There is a desire to involve as many people and perspectives as

---

[5]"Plain language" is a term used to describe communication written and designed so people can understand information that is important to their lives.

possible. Obtaining additional input from employers and payers would strengthen HLI. In terms of sustainability, core funding is needed. The principles of quality, safety, cost containment, health disparities reduction, and patient-centered care resonate very well with stakeholders, Abrams said. For any organization, there is always the question of whether the organization should go public and incrementally build capacity, or alternatively, build capacity first and then launch programs. Abrams said that HLI continues to develop its own skill sets and emerge as an independent entity.

DISCUSSION

As a member of the U.S. Pharmacopeia (USP) Health Literacy Advisory Committee, roundtable member Cindy Brach asked Silberman about the lack of progress made on prescription drug labeling in North Carolina. She asked how the NC Board of Pharmacy was approached, what resistance to labeling reform was expressed, and whether having a USP standard would be helpful. Brach clarified that the federal government has no authority over regulating prescription drug labels and that it is left up to state boards. She added that the USP Advisory Committee will be publishing a standard in the form of a chapter on a patient-centered prescription labeling.[6]

Silberman replied that the NC Board of Pharmacy had not been included on their task force. Pharmacists were on the task force, but not the board. The board was asked to make a presentation to the task force when prescription labeling was recognized as an important issue. There is interest in the issue, but Silberman speculated that the Board of Pharmacy might be concerned about the reaction of local pharmacies to any labeling changes. She added that having nationally recognized guidelines would be very helpful. A standard would prevent local boards from having to develop their own labeling guidelines. Movement on the part of state boards may depend on individual personalities and their interest in taking this on. Brach mentioned that California has implemented labeling reforms. Silberman said that if other states have already adopted new standards, then North Carolina might be willing to reexamine their position.

Brach was very interested in Silberman's discussion of the role of malpractice insurance carriers in promoting health literacy. She asked

---

[6]The USP published recommendations for prescriptions medication labels in May, 2010. The recommendations formed the basis for a draft chapter that was circulated in early 2011 for comment. At the time of the writing of this report, a final version of the chapter has not been released.

Silberman to provide some detail on their engagement and whether or not they are offering any kind of incentives for health literacy training. Silberman said that malpractice carriers were not part of the task force and probably should have been. They were invited to participate when the task force decided that a recommendation in this area should be considered. In addition, NC Medical Mutual agreed to write an article for the state medical journal about their interest in health literacy (Hickson and Jenkins, 2007). Silberman said that she was not sure if the insurer was offering an incentive for health literacy training. The insurer is aware of, and letting its subscribers know about, the research that shows that physicians are more likely to be sued for malpractice if they have poor patient communication skills. NC Medical Mutual has developed a training toolkit that includes a section on the informed consent process in the context of risk management. This toolkit is used in the provider training.

Carla Funk, executive director of the Medical Library Association, commented that health sciences librarians and librarians in general are available as collaborators and partners in health literacy initiatives. She added that librarians have valuable experience in working with and educating health care providers. The Medical Library Association has developed a health literacy tutorial through a contract from the National Library of Medicine. The tutorial and a curriculum are freely available to all health care providers and librarians. Abrams agreed that librarians are crucial for progress to be made on health literacy and mentioned the productive collaboration between Health Literacy Iowa and the health sciences librarian at the University of Iowa.

Roundtable member Benard Dreyer asked the panelists to describe how they were able to engage the parties needed to make progress in health literacy, for example, the health department and the payers. He observed that having stakeholders take responsibility is a key to sustainability. Abrams responded that in Iowa some of the key stakeholders had already become involved in health literacy. She found that establishing personal relationships and sharing local data and stories are key to making connections with decision makers. She mentioned that in Iowa, the director of the Department of Public Health has been very supportive. Progress with the Department of Education has not been as great, probably because of the many competing demands faced by the department. Abrams pointed out that a strong business case, economic analyses, and the opportunities provided by healthcare reform could provide some leverage to promote health literacy.

Silberman added that a challenge faced when working with stakeholders is that when they leave their positions, there is a loss of an educated leader within their organization. North Carolina has had the advantage of having stable leadership within the Medicaid managed-care Program,

Community Care of NC. However, there has been turnover in the position of Assistant Secretary for the Department of Health and Human Services. This meant that a reeducation process had to be undertaken. Silberman mentioned that North Carolina is fortunate in having national experts in health literacy who are able to share the results of their research and engage key stakeholders.

Roundtable member Will Ross pointed out the importance of targeting health literacy interventions to schools, especially students from kindergarten through grade 12. He asked the panelists to discuss barriers to engaging state departments of education in health literacy initiatives. Abrams indicated that progress is being made in Iowa. For example, a core curriculum that includes life skills for the 21st century has been developed, and health literacy is one of the four key focus areas. In addition, the Department of Education supports the New Readers of Iowa program and an early child literacy program called Reach Out and Read. Abrams observed that while these are encouraging steps, a greater level of communication between the education and health sectors would be desirable as there are many more opportunities to explore.

Silberman stated that the North Carolina task force did not include kindergarten through grade 12 education. However, the task force did work with the Department of Public Instruction on health issues. Health literacy is in the core curriculum, but she indicated that one problem is that the core curriculum is only a recommended curriculum. The decision on using it is left to each local education agency. Silberman added that the standardized tests that are given at the end of the year do not include health literacy. This means that the subject is likely not given much coverage in the curriculum. That said, some schools are doing a good job, but on a statewide level, progress is needed. To keep this in context, Silberman mentioned the great challenges in keeping students in school until they graduate. For teachers, this is a priority.

Roundtable member Patrick McGarry asked the panelists if there are any performance measures related to health literacy applied to states, and if there are such measures, how states are performing. Silberman replied that there are no statewide performance measures. However, in North Carolina, periodic reviews are conducted on the status of the NCIOM's Task Force on Health Literacy recommendations. She mentioned the existence of performance measures related to chronic disease management in the state's Medicaid program. These health outcomes measures are contingent, in part, on how effectively health care professionals communicate with their patients. Abrams pointed out how important it is to understand the validity of performance measures. For example, one of the Centers for Medicare and Medicaid Services (CMS) core measures for heart failure is whether the provider has discussed the various components of discharge planning. A provider may check a box indicating that he or she has provided information, but it is not really clear whether the patient understood the information given. Abrams indicated that this is what should be measured in terms of health literacy.

George Isham, roundtable chair, asked whether health literacy was being measured statewide, and if a measure of population health literacy is informative. Abrams and Silberman both stated that they have not made such a measurement in either Iowa or North Carolina. Silberman discussed the research conducted at the University of North Carolina on the effect of health literacy interventions on health outcomes among people with different levels of health literacy. That research found, for both diabetes and congestive heart failure, that health literacy interventions improved outcomes for everyone, but that improvements were greater for people with low health literacy. Silberman went on to discuss the issue of the universality of low health literacy and how low health literacy can be experienced by almost everyone in given circumstances. She described her experience of taking her mother who was dying of cancer from the hospital to her home. The discharging physician gave her instructions for home care, and she wrote them down. However, when she got home, her notes were indecipherable. This is just another example of the importance for clinicians to always be clear, always communicate well, and to always have materials that are understandable. Silberman pointed out that the AHRQ commercials on health literacy use this universal precaution model to encourage people to ask questions and feel comfortable so they can become informed. Abrams added that changing and improving the health literacy of the entire population is a huge undertaking and likely very difficult to measure. She felt that such measurement will need to be investigated and may represent a long-term goal.

Reggie Cayetano, UCLA Division of Cancer Prevention and Control, asked Silberman how the North Carolina Task Force has addressed the needs of the state's Asian and Hispanic populations in terms of health literacy. Silberman mentioned that because the Asian population is not sizable in North Carolina, most of the task force's attention has been directed to the state's Hispanic population, which is expanding rapidly. She mentioned that between 1990 and 2000, North Carolina had the fastest growing Hispanic population in the United States. Silberman indicated that although some programs are in place, more work is needed. For example, there are bilingual staff within the Medicaid networks and community health centers, but there are no certified interpreters. A center is working with the AHEC program to train interpreters, but an impediment to placing them in clinical environments is lack of reimbursement for interpreter services. The importance of having both trained interpreters and people who have cultural competence is recognized, but more resources are needed to facilitate progress in these areas.

THE MISSOURI EXPERIENCE

Arthur Culbert, Ph.D.
Health Literacy Missouri

Health Literacy Missouri (HLM) was founded as an independent 501(c)(3) center in 2009 with support from the Missouri Foundation for Health. The center's mission is to improve the health status of Missouri residents through health literacy. The center creates health information products that are understandable and widely available with the aim of empowering individuals and promoting positive changes in behaviors. HLM functions to create systematic change in provider-patient encounters, to offer education resources that help providers communicate effectively with patients, and to provide access to plain language health care information.

A six-minute video about HLM demonstrated the need for health literacy interventions.[7] According to Culbert, an estimated 1.6 million Missouri residents have trouble reading prescriptions labels, following medical instructions, and filling out medical-related forms. The costs associated with poor health literacy can be counted not only in terms of pain and suffering, he said, but also in financial terms, estimated to total $3.3 to $7.5 billion annually for Missouri residents. Health literacy is viewed as critical to address the state's poor performance on health indicators. Missouri ranks in the bottom quartile of U.S. states in terms of smoking, obesity, and diabetes prevalence. The state ranks last in terms of state funding for public health. The state has a large rural population, which means that health-related messages have to be targeted to residents of less populated areas. The video illustrated several of the literacy center's programs including those targeted to language minorities (e.g., Spanish, Chinese), adult learners, and school groups. In addition to these consumer groups, clinicians have been engaged in educational programs to improve patient-provider communications. Motivating changes in health behavior can best be accomplished through activities like these, implemented at the community and state level, Culbert said.

One of the challenges in Missouri is that large areas of the state are either not served, or are underserved, by broadband Internet coverage. Yet public health communications are key. Consequently, HLM has pri-

---

[7]The video is available at http://www.healthliteracymissouri.org/ (accessed February 7, 2011).

oritized implementing interventions within the healthcare system. Integrating health literacy into ongoing related programs such as programs to reduce medical errors has been a fruitful approach. Stand-alone health literacy programs are not nearly as powerful, Culbert said.

Collaboration and the ability to connect with partners are a particular strength of HLM. The program attempts to quickly translate the lessons of research into best practices. HLM has worked effectively with academic partners (e.g., the University of Missouri, St. Louis University, Washington University in St. Louis, Missouri State University) and all of the state's AHECs. Over its first 3 years of operation, HLM identified the needs of the state's population and developed a logic model with which to plan intervention strategies. Effective working relationships developed because stakeholders were able to work collaboratively.

With support from the Missouri Foundation for Health, HLM is active in 84 of the state's 112 counties. The center worked with Dr. Nicole Lurie to develop geographic information system (GIS) mapping software to identify areas in the state with large numbers of people with low health literacy. An estimate was made of the financial costs of low health literacy in Missouri with the help of John Vernon who had just completed a national report on this topic. Another first step for the center was to field test the *Living with Diabetes Manual* developed by Mike Wolf and Dean Schillinger. The center has also helped distribute a popular online health literacy magazine aimed at high school students. The magazine, called *Youmagazine* (Youmagazine.net) has been made available in 29 Missouri schools. Finally, the Universal Precautions Toolkit[8] developed in North Carolina with support from AHRQ has been central in efforts to engage the community around health literacy.

HLM's grassroots activities have been supported by 31 demonstration grant programs implemented in 84 Missouri counties. These projects are viewed as incubators of change and are diverse in terms of their scope and audience. They cover programs targeted by age (e.g., youth, the elderly) and by population subgroup (e.g., Bosnians, Chinese, African Americans, Hispanics). HLM's goal is to identify interventions that work and then replicate them. The programs have been sequenced to start at different times. Some of them are completing their first 2 years, allowing for lessons learned to be applied elsewhere.

The center has worked with the state's four medical schools (three

---

[8]"Universal precautions" refers to taking specific actions that minimize risk for everyone when it is unclear which patients may be affected. For example, health care workers take universal precautions when they minimize the risk of blood-borne disease by using gloves and proper disposal techniques. Health literacy universal precautions are needed because providers don't always know which patients have limited health literacy (http://www.ahrq.gov/qual/literacy/, accessed February 7, 2011).

allopathic, one osteopathic) to develop three unique programs. This first one, *Straight Talk With Your Doc* is a simulation where medical students and other health professionals volunteer to play the role of a provider, usually a doctor, and teach their clients how to be empowered to engage successfully with the healthcare system. The experience thus far has been very positive and it is being translated into multiple languages. The second program, *The Standardized Patient* is targeted to medical students. The third program is a *Practice Improvement Module* that has been approved by the American Academy of Internal Medicine and will be available for those who are securing or maintaining their licensure.

Rewriting materials using plain language is a major function of HLM. HLM has worked with drug companies, insurance agencies, and hospitals to improve their materials. The center is working on a pricing scheme so clients can be billed.

Rima Rudd from the Harvard School of Public Health serves as the senior advisor to HLM and has helped the center address issues relating to hospital health literacy assessments, facility signage, patient information materials, and patient healthcare system navigation. Barnes-Jewish Hospital, the largest employer in the state, has engaged the center to help redesign its ambulatory care centers. The clinics will be health literacy friendly. This means that visitors will understand the signage, staff will be trained, and patient education materials will be understandable.

Educating the business community on the costs associated with limited health literacy is a very important area, Culbert said, as is the need to engage political stakeholders. Missouri Governor Nixon's designation of October as health literacy month is an achievement in the political area. Health literacy is not a partisan issue. People are able to disassociate the issue from the debate over healthcare reform and focus on the cost of low health literacy, both in terms of actual dollars as well as in emotional and health terms. The center has been working with the governor and his staff to facilitate the adoption of electronic health records. A consumer engagement committee will be involved with decisions regarding written materials, public service announcements, and other implementation activities.

There is growing interest in health literacy across the entire health care spectrum. Enthusiasm across the state is evident from a stakeholder summit held June 2010 that attracted over 250 people. The creation of a nationwide network of state health literacy centers has been proposed. Several states in the Midwest (Iowa, Minnesota, Missouri, and Wisconsin) began meeting together in 2008. The meetings have been instrumental in sharing best practices and providing mutual support.

The online activities are expanding, Culbert said. In its first year of operation the HLM website logged more than 100,000 visits to the site. Culbert speculated that the main reason for the site's popularity is that the site houses a collection of more than 10,000 health literacy resources, including toolkits. The online library also includes almost 200 videos related to health literacy. The center benefits from a full-time digital librarian who researches source materials.

While the center continues to rely on hard-copy communications including newspapers, it has branched out into the world of social media including Twitter and Facebook. The center uses LinkedIn, a professional social networking medium, to get information to physicians. Flickr is used to store pictures from all of the center's events, and Vimeo is used to house the video collection. Delicious is a site where individuals can find the most bookmarked organizations websites for a given topic. The center also hosts a blog, with Helen Osborne as the first guest blogger. In October 2010, the center participated in the health literacy Twitter town hall hosted by Cynthia Baur, CDC's Senior Health Literacy Advisor, and by the Department of Health and Human Services' healthfinder.gov team. A few weeks later, HLM hosted a Twitter town hall where 92 people joined in the conversation. This venue has allowed the center to expand its reach to new audiences.

Culbert concluded his presentation by reviewing some of HLM's successes and challenges. One indicator of success is the wide coverage received following the release of 26 HLM press releases. The releases delivered at the local level have generated 280 newspaper stories that have an estimated readership of one million. Print media remains very important, especially in rural areas with poor broadband coverage. A remaining challenge is how best to develop models of community engagement appropriate for the unique needs of rural and urban areas. Evaluations of HLM's activities will make a contribution to the literature and body of evidence regarding the role of states in advancing health literacy, Culbert concluded.

LOUISIANA STATEWIDE HEALTH LITERACY INITIATIVE

Terry Davis, Ph.D.
Louisiana State University Health Sciences Center Shreveport

Davis began her presentation by acknowledging State Senator Lydia Jackson for her active involvement in Louisiana's health literacy initiatives and for her assistance in crafting the IOM workshop presentation. She pointed out that involving political leaders at the state level is important because with healthcare reform, states will enroll more people in Medicaid and yet have fewer resources as a result of hiring freezes and budget cuts. There will be difficulties in assisting people as they enroll in Medicaid. In addition, more information and services will have to be computer based, which can be problematic for people with low literacy. According to a recent IOM report, 96 percent of states have simplified enrollment forms and 82 percent of states offer one-on-one assistance (Somers and Mahadevan, 2010); but despite these efforts, more than 80 percent of uninsured African-American children and 70 percent of uninsured Hispanic children who are eligible for Medicaid or the Children's Health Insurance Program (CHIP) are not enrolled. Even though enrollment has been simplified, these figures indicate that more work is needed. States play an important role in making healthcare information and services user friendly.

With implementation of health care reform and the Plain Language Act,[9] there is a greater need for states to focus on health literacy, Davis said. All states must enroll beneficiaries under age 65 with incomes of up to 133 percent of the federal poverty level. This is going to greatly expand enrollment. In 2007 there were 58 million enrollees. By 2014 one-quarter of U.S. residents will be enrolled in Medicaid. With healthcare reform, Louisiana is expected to enroll 384,000 new Medicaid beneficiaries and the size of the uninsured population is expected to drop by 50 to 75 percent.

Davis reviewed the history of the Louisiana Statewide Health Literacy Initiative that had its beginnings in 2002. As Davis and Senator Jackson began to envision a health literacy initiative they considered the following questions:

- What is possible?
- What first steps should be taken?
- Who should be involved?
- How do you reach community leaders?
- How do you approach legislators, the secretary of health, and the governor?
- How do you inform decision makers about the cost of low health literacy, and how health literacy impacts cost and quality?
- What do you ask of policy makers? What specifically is being asked of them?
- How can health and education groups across the state be engaged?
- How can a statewide health literacy group be organized with sufficient representation, yet remain small enough to achieve consensus and accomplish tasks?
- How can the process and planned programs be financially supported?

---

[9]The Plain Language Act of 2010 requires the federal government to write all new publications, forms, and publicly distributed documents in a "clear, concise, well-organized" manner that follows the best practices of plain language writing. See www.plainlanguage.gov (accessed February 7, 2011).

In Louisiana, it was unclear whether the legislature would allocate scarce funds to train health professionals and educators to improve oral and written communication, particularly communication to help people better navigate the system, be healthier, and manage chronic disease.

Louisiana has a unique landscape, distinct culture, and rich heritage. Davis said. Most families have lived in the state for generations and are rooted in their communities. Louisiana is ranked as the unhealthiest state in the nation. There are high rates of uninsured individuals and a low-performing healthcare delivery system. The state has the highest public healthcare cost with the worst outcomes. One-third of children live in poverty. Nearly half of ninth graders do not graduate from high school in 4 years. According to the 1993 National Adult Literacy Survey (NALS), approximately 28 percent of adults in Louisiana ranked in the lowest literacy level. On a positive note, Davis cited Louisiana's long history of charity health care. In the 1930s, 10 state hospitals were designated to care for the poor. These hospitals were not, however, set up to provide easy access to preventive and primary care.

It is key, Davis said, to identify a health literacy champion in the state legislature. The legislative champion should have an interest in both education and health and have a legislative record in these areas. She also suggested that the champion be able to conceptually link health and literacy and education. In her view, the champion must also be skilled in connecting existing health and education officials. Strong critical thinking and problem solving skills, good communication skills, an ability to collaborate and get things done, and knowledge of who the key "go-to" people are to open doors are also important attributes of a champion.

In Louisiana, Senator Lydia Jackson has championed health literacy initiatives. Since being elected to the House of Representatives in 1999, Senator Jackson has developed a reputation as an effective, hardworking, and innovative legislator. She quickly assesses what is going on, listens more than she talks, and has a knack for figuring out what is possible and what is not possible. Her accomplishments led to her election to the Senate. She is viewed as a leader in the legislature and a champion of healthcare issues. One of the ways Senator Jackson became interested in health is through her attendance at Davis's grand rounds at the medical school. Other community leaders have been invited to attend grand rounds as well as other presentations at the medical school. Subsequently, Senator Jackson invited Davis to speak at some town hall meetings. One of those meetings had every regional legislator present.

In 2003 the legislature passed a law to establish a health literacy task force. To facilitate passage, Senator Jackson identified key legislators and committees to contact. Davis addressed key decision makers and showed a videotape featuring people struggling with healthcare tasks. The message resonated with the legislature. The legislation created an Interagency Task Force on Health Literacy. Although no funding was attached, support was located to employ a part-time administrative assistant. The task force initially included 31 members from 23 health and education organizations across the state. It's responsibilities were as follows:

- Study the health literacy of Louisiana residents.
- Identify groups at risk for low health literacy.
- Identify barriers to accessing services and communicating with providers.
- Make recommendations to
  o improve health literacy,
  o promote providers' use of plain language,
  o simplify forms and procedures,
  o develop easy to understand health info,
  o develop health literacy curricula, and
  o examine impact on quality and cost.

The law mandated that the heads of different organizations and agencies be contacted to select a representative. For example, the U.S. Department of Agriculture (USDA) was invited to participate because it has an interest in health literacy, especially as it relates to obesity. Davis described the USDA as a wonderful partner, in part because it has cooperative extensions in every U.S. county. The task force met every 6 weeks in Baton Rouge. Davis served with co-chairman Sheila Chauvin, head of medical education and research at Louisiana State University Health Sciences Center in New Orleans. The face-to-face meetings fostered trust, collaboration, and a sense of confidence that something could be accomplished statewide to improve health and health communication.

A needs assessment was the task force's first task. A literature review and a survey of health and education organizations and state agencies were conducted. Relevant materials were posted to a website. A medical librarian on the task force was instrumental in identifying relevant resources. There appeared to be very little, or no, interagency coordination. And in 2004 when this work was initiated, there was little awareness of health literacy. When health literacy activities were identified, they usually represented the work of impassioned advocates working within silos. The needs assessment, completed in 2005, identified several problems:

- Medicaid applicants struggled with instructions that were too long, confusing, and difficult to complete.
- Individuals calling to renew enrollment in CHIP had difficulties. One in three persons calling for assistance talked to someone who

could not answer their questions. Many callers were put on hold for over 10 minutes or got repeated busy signals.
- Many citizens lacked the knowledge and skill to adequately manage chronic disease, or to use preventive services.
- Louisiana schools of medicine, nursing, pharmacy, and public health did not have a health literacy curriculum.
- Health education is required in schools grades kindergarten to grade 9, but in 2005, the content did not adequately provide students with basic health knowledge and skills. The Department of Education was very interested in revamping the curricula.
- There was inadequate health education content in adult literacy classes.

One of the early health literacy accomplishments in Louisiana was the development of a proposal to provide "train the trainer" workshops based on the American Medical Association model. The plan was to use online modules to train 7,000 healthcare professional staff and educators to communicate more effectively. The proposal also included the development of user-friendly materials and forms. Participation was to be tracked, the training content reviewed, and the outcome of the training evaluated. As the proposal was being finalized however, hurricanes Katrina and Rita hit. Commerce in New Orleans was virtually eliminated and about half of sales tax revenue was lost. There were only two hospitals open 6 months after the hurricanes. Doctors' offices and most hospitals had lost all their medical records. The Department of Veterans Affairs had fortunately transitioned to an electronic medical record system. Louisiana is still recovering, and public education in New Orleans, which was one of the worst in the country, is now doing better, in part, because of the Teach for America program.

Davis mentioned that the IOM workshop in Los Angeles has served to reunite her with Senator Jackson to strategize on statewide initiatives on health literacy. With a commitment to integrate health literacy within the existing delivery system, there is hope that progress can be made without a large financial investment. Advocates of health literacy at the state level should, Davis concluded, find a legislative champion; connect with key health and education officials; develop a plan to make state health information and services easier to understand and act upon; integrate the plan into the existing delivery system; partner to make the case that improving health literacy is good public policy, reduces cost, and improves quality; and propose a realistic funding level for a legislature with a shrinking budget.

DISCUSSION

Roundtable member Winston Wong asked Culbert how health literacy might ultimately improve population outcomes such as obesity and how the Missouri initiative has addressed obesity, both in the short- and long-term. Culbert responded by pointing out the importance of health literacy as a social determinant of health. In Missouri, the aim is to try to create information that helps people understand why they should be making changes to address their particular problem in their particular situation. The strategy in Missouri is not to mandate behavior change, but rather to motivate individuals within communities. Five- and 10-year goals are being established.

Health Literacy Missouri is piloting a *Living with Diabetes* guide and plans to focus attention on chronic diseases. Providing programs in schools and targeting new mothers and children may be key to taking a prevention approach that is directed to the next generation. Davis added that incentives may be key to motivating both providers and consumers to participate in new initiatives and change their behaviors. Wong suggested that health literacy is often considered in the context of a specific clinical encounter. He noted how interesting it is to think of obesity as an epidemic or disease state that can be influenced by health literacy efforts statewide. Davis mentioned in response that the USDA is sponsoring a $25 million program to address obesity and health literacy.

Gloria Mayer, Institute for Healthcare Advancement (IHA), asked Culbert whether the state health literacy initiative has addressed the needs of nursing students. She pointed out the important role of nurses in hospitals and outpatient clinics in providing education and counseling to patients. In her experience, relatively few nurses attend IHA health literacy conferences. Culbert responded that nurses in Missouri have been quick to recognize the importance of health literacy and have been enthusiastic supporters of the program. Nurse educators have been incorporating health literacy throughout their curriculum and creating learning opportunities for trainees.

Davis added that according to her focus group research, nurses consider communication a part of their mission. Doctors often view diagnosis and the development of a treatment plan as their main mission. In some ways then, nurses could be considered an easier group to partner with. Many times they are the ones that are most receptive to health literacy messages and to act on them.

Leonard and Cecelia Doak of Patient Learning Associates, Inc., commended the presenters for using pictures and video to effectively communicate the health literacy story to legislators and to the general public. Pictures, and the stories that accompany them, can be more powerful than words. Davis agreed and added that pictures of real people have an emotional impact that elicits responses. For a new guide being developed on heart disease, images of patients and their families in their homes and places of business are being used. It is important to impart the message that health affects the entire family.

Roundtable member Will Ross asked Culbert and Davis if the regional initiatives they had undertaken were effective. He pointed out that states have become great incubators for developing innovative and effective programs. Ross asked if there was a strategic plan for their expansion. He mentioned the importance of identifying leaders in other states that had not quite matured in the development of statewide health literacy initiatives.

Culbert described the benefits of cross-state collaboration and how his program has been enriched by the experiences of others in the Midwest. He identified the important role of providing technical assistance to interested states. As an example, he mentioned a contact he made through the National Institute For Literacy (NIFL) email list. An individual from Pennsylvania was interested in hosting a literacy summit and was looking for guidance. Culbert was able to provide assistance and Pennsylvania subsequently held a very successful summit bringing together interested stakeholders. Health Literacy Missouri is seeking funding to improve its ability to offer technical assistance. HLM staff will continue to attend national meetings and while there provide assistance to interested state representatives. Culbert indicated that having someone at the state level to organize and coordinate ongoing activities would be very helpful.

Davis discussed three factors that are motivating organizations to address health literacy. First, hospitals and other health care facilities are making efforts to adhere to the Joint Commission's health literacy communication (The Joint Commission, 2007, 2008). Second, the CDC is supporting public health departments with training opportunities and guidance on health marketed to assist them as they integrate health literacy into their programming (http://www.cdc.gov/healthmarketing/health literacy/, accessed February 9, 2011). Finally, AHRQ and the National Institutes of Health (NIH) are driving research in this area (http://www.ahrq.gov/browse/hlitix.htm, accessed February 9, 2011; http://www.nih.gov/icd/od/ocpl/resources/healthliteracyresearch.htm, accessed February 9, 2011). Davis added that some state-level activities emerge from the efforts of a single impassioned leader.

Roundtable chairperson Isham asked the panel how the IOM's Roundtable on Health Literacy might foster progress at the state level. Culbert indicated that the IOM's powerful voice is very helpful in advocating for health literacy at the national level. However, in his opinion, the biggest successes around health care have come at the state and community level. Davis added that the IOM's 2004 report was instrumental in calling attention to health literacy (IOM, 2004). At this point, the roundtable might focus on the implications of health reform. For example, one-fourth of the U.S. population will be enrolled in Medicaid. The materials for enrollment and other information must be improved so they are easier to access and understand. Another area in need of attention is pharmaceutical use, improving the public's understanding of how to take prescription and over-the-counter medicines safely.

Julie Kwan, National Network of Libraries of Medicine, provided information on the National Library of Medicine's release of documentation on how to connect an electronic health record through a patient portal to MedlinePlus (http://www.nlm.nih.gov/medlineplus/, accessed February 9, 2011). The service is available in English and Spanish at no cost. Patients will be able to search for information on medical conditions and medications. MedlinePlus includes pictures and videos that may be particularly useful for those with low literacy. Culbert discussed the importance of libraries in the health literacy movement. Health Literacy Missouri has worked with librarians to create a list of suggested health literacy holdings. As local libraries in Missouri purchase their books, there will be a whole set of recommended health literacy books that will go on the shelves.

Kelli Ham, National Network of Libraries of Medicine, described her involvement with the California State Library in the publication of a toolkit for public librarians. The toolkit helps local librarians provide quality health information services. It was developed for California, but it has been widely disseminated across the country. Culbert added that the United Kingdom has been running a health literacy program for the past decade from libraries. He suggested that there is much to be learned from this approach. Libraries should be one of the first venues to think about in advancing health literacy.

Shanpin Fanchiang, an educator at Rancho Los Amigos National Rehabilitation Center, asked the panel how to approach legislators at both the state and federal level to ensure that health literacy becomes a part of all healthcare professionals' licensing and reaccreditation. She emphasized how important it is for healthcare workers to have a basic understanding of health literacy and how to incorporate it into their practice. Davis suggested identifying state legislators with a health and education track record and inviting them to a facility so they can experience the consequences of poor communication and low literacy. Begin to develop a relationship with legislative representatives so they will begin to see how they can help address issues through state policy. Davis also suggested working with the professional organizations representing physicians, nurses, pharmacists, and others to address accreditation issues. She discussed her unsuccessful attempt to interest the National Boards of

Medicine in adding health literacy topics to exams. In terms of maximizing education and training opportunities, Davis recommended embedding health literacy into regular curriculum content rather than presenting it as a stand-alone topic. Isham added that national professional organizations often set general policy, but that licensure and accreditation for most professionals is at the state level. Therefore, a two-level strategy could be considered. Culbert referred to the national discussion underway about core health professional competencies and educational reform. The Federation of Associations of Schools of the Health Professions (FASHP) is addressing this issue with a focus on cross-disciplinary education, he said.

4

The Role of the University in Improving States' Health Literacy

HOW THE UNIVERSITY CAN ADVANCE STATE HEALTH LITERACY

Dean Schillinger, M.D.
University of California, San Francisco

Schillinger reviewed the seven goals of the 2010 Department of Health and Human Services (HHS) National Action Plan to Improve Health Literacy. He then described examples of community-engaged research that improve the health literacy of the state's population at the University of California, San Francisco (UCSF) and at other health sciences campuses in California. The UC campuses are a resource for training the future healthcare workforce, for providing clinical care, innovating care, advancing public policy, and conducting impactful research.

The seven goals of the National Action Plan to Improve Health Literacy are to (HHS, 2010)

1. develop and disseminate health and safety information that is accurate, accessible, and actionable;
2. promote changes in the healthcare system that improve health information, communication, informed decision making, and access to health services;
3. incorporate accurate, standards-based, and developmentally appropriate health and science information and curricula in child care and education through the university level;

4. support and expand local efforts to provide adult education, English language instruction, and culturally and linguistically appropriate health information services in the community;
5. build partnerships, develop guidance, and change policies;
6. increase basic research and the development, implementation, and evaluation of practices and interventions to improve health literacy; and
7. increase the dissemination and use of evidence-based health literacy practices and interventions.

Research on health literacy can be viewed as translational research. The National Institutes of Health (NIH) has in the last few years revisited its mission and has focused on developing expertise and products in translational research, moving from bench to bedside, and then from bedside to community. Over the past half century NIH primarily funded Translational 1 (T-1) research, which is research on "the transfer of new understandings of disease mechanisms gained in the laboratory into the development of new methods for diagnosis, therapy, and prevention and their first testing in humans" (Sung et al., 2003). Translational 2 (T-2) research involves bedside-to-community research, as does some Transitional 3 (T-3) research, which is defined as "the translation of results from clinical studies into everyday clinical practice and health decision making" (Sung et al., 2003). Much effort has been put into T-1 discovery. While the gap in funding between T-1 and T-2 research is immense, increased attention is now being paid to how T-1 discoveries can be incorporated into clinical and public health practice to promote behavior change and reduce health disparities. Unfortunately, the results of bench research do not spontaneously diffuse throughout the practice community. For example, the findings from randomized controlled trials may not affect community practices for years to decades. The Clinical Translational Science Awards from the NIH are accelerating the pace of discovery from the bench all the way to population health, Schillinger said.

The UCSF received an NIH Translational Sciences Award and established the Clinical and Translational Science Institute (CTSI). CTSI challenges, encourages, and supports UCSF researchers to take the research capital at UCSF—the great wealth of clinical research discoveries, knowledge, and know-how—and link it with community partners' expertise and priorities to effectively translate research into interventions that can be scaled to make a measurable impact on the health of the local community and eliminate disparities. CTSI has developed four working principles. These are as follows:

1. Take a population health perspective.
2. Invest in community partnerships.
3. Require transdisciplinary science.
4. Translation is itself a subject matter for research.

While there are outstanding schools of medicine, nursing, pharmacy, and dentistry at UCSF, there is no school of communication or a school of education, thereby hampering efforts to involve those disciplines in research, Schillinger said. There are, however, pockets of expertise in these areas, and collaboration with investigators at the University of California, Berkeley, for example, help fill these transdisciplinary gaps.

A transdisciplinary research approach would ideally involve such fields as epidemiology, biomedical science and technology, behavioral science, psychology, communication and information technology, political science, sociology, cognitive science, social marketing, and economics. These fields are integral to understanding the ecological model for health. This model assumes that many factors affect individual health and that individuals can be considered to be striving for health and the maintenance of health in the context of multiple environmental influences from the family all the way up to local and national political decisions.

CTSI is committed to the notion that translation is itself a subject matter for research. There is a science to dissemination and a science to implementation. Schillinger pointed out that in such research, an emphasis on external validity sometimes comes at the expense of internal validity. The methodology underpinning the controlled clinical trial often dictates that a narrowly defined set of people be included in the trial. Many times individuals are excluded from participation if they are not within certain age ranges or have comorbid health conditions. The clinical trial may be internally valid insofar as it advances our understanding of important questions for those groups represented in the trial, but it may have little relevance to the real-world patients in real-world settings. Schillinger suggested that a balance must be struck; that is, the representativeness of study samples, the study settings, and the study interventions as they relate to the real world all need to be attended to, while also trying to maximize internal validity.

Schillinger cited the work of Lawrence Green, who through his work at the Centers for Disease Control and Prevention (CDC) and the National Cancer Institute, has eloquently and persistently advocated for the need not only to put research into practice, but to also "put practice back into research." This principle has been at the heart of the primary care practice-based research networks that have engaged community settings in framing research questions, designing interventions that are feasible, and testing them in the real world. This approach, if expanded beyond primary care research, would represent a sea change for research institutions such as UCSF.

UCSF has used this community-based approach, for example, in researching the role of chronic hepatitis B on the development of hepatocellular cancer. Chronic hepatitis B-related cancer is a leading cause of cancer deaths among Asian and Pacific Islanders in the San Francisco Bay Area. Fundamental clinical and epidemiologic research has been conducted on hepatocellular carcinoma, surveillance, screening, and antiviral treatments, but high rates of infection and cancer death have persisted. With the leadership of Dr. Tung Nguyen, CTSI has linked researchers and clinicians with public health advocates and community members to try to address these epidemics. To further public awareness, social marketing campaigns among the Asian and Pacific Islander community in the San Francisco Bay Area have emerged to promote testing, vaccination, and treatment.

Schillinger provided another example of research at UCSF related to health literacy, health promotion, and health communication, research that is in response to the first goal of the National Action Plan to Improve Health Literacy. With support from the Agency for Healthcare Research and Quality (AHRQ), medication summary guides are being developed for vulnerable populations with rheumatoid arthritis (RA) (Edward Yelin is the principal investigator [PI]). In describing the context for the study, Schillinger discussed how the treatment of RA has advanced greatly over the last decade. A number of new biologic therapies are remarkably effective if prescribed to the patient early in the disease course. These medications can change the trajectory of the disease such that people are much less likely to be disabled from RA than they were 15 years ago. Yet the medications are very costly and have to be taken exactly as prescribed. There can be serious side effects if too much medication is taken, there is a narrow therapeutic window in terms of dosage, and monitoring for adverse events is critical. To be effective, patients must be extremely involved in their medication management and care. Descriptive studies have shown that there are significant sociodemographic disparities in the degree to which patients receive these highly effective treatments. The investigators have hypothesized and shown that health communication is one of the contributors to these disparities. Box 4-1 presents the study objectives, and Box 4-2 lists the anticipated outcomes of the study.

Another example of UCSF research is the Bay Area Breast Cancer and the Environment Research Program (Robert Hiatt, PI) which involves basic, applied, and community-based approaches. There are three core projects:

1. Environmental Influences and the Windows of Susceptibility in Breast Cancer Risk Project—NCI funded, a highly technical project that includes T-1 research
2. Early Environmental Exposures and Human Puberty Project, conducted in collaboration with investigators at Kaiser Permanente
3. Community Outreach and Translation Core, in collaboration with Zero Breast Cancer, a community-based advocacy organization

The context for the program is the observation of a trend that puberty is occurring at younger ages among girls. Because early onset of puberty is a risk factor for breast cancer, there is interest in whether early exposure to certain environmental chemicals, obesity, genetics, and other factors raise the risk of early puberty. There are tremendous challenges associated with communicating to the public about findings related to environmental toxins, their association with early puberty, and their potential relationship to breast cancer risk. There is need for communication across disciplines, among biologists, physical scientists, biochemists, community members,

---

BOX 4-1
Study Objectives

- Assess the knowledge of RA therapies among vulnerable populations and the utility of current RA summary guides.
- Develop print and video adaptations of guides and a decision aid tool.
- Conduct a pilot trial to test adapted guides and the decision aid, and evaluate the impact of tools on outcomes.

SOURCE: Schillinger, 2010.

BOX 4-2
Anticipated Study Outcomes

- A low literacy, plain language, medication summary guide in English, Spanish, and Chinese for vulnerable populations with RA.
- A decision aid tool derived from the adapted medication summary guide to improve patient-physician communication, reduce decisional conflict, and improve adherence and outcomes in RA patients with limited health literacy.

SOURCE: Schillinger, 2010.

and advocates. The program has created opportunities and products (The Breast Biologues, bayrea.bcerc.org/cotcpubs) that communicate findings to these various constituencies. It is a model that can be replicated for a number of diseases and conditions.

In response to the second goal of the National Action Plan to Improve Health Literacy, Schillinger described an AHRQ-funded project to provide automated telephone self-management (ATSM) support for patients with diabetes (Dean Schillinger, PI). The project involves the use of a simple technology, automated telephone support, to provide patients with a basic understanding of diabetes and access to self-management tools and support. It is an interactive health technology relying on touchtone telephones. The service places a call to patients weekly, and recorded messages are in the patient's native language: English, Spanish, or Chinese. If the patient reports an episode of hypoglycemia or low blood sugar, he or she will get a call back from a nurse. If a patient reports that everything is going well, that he or she is not smoking, that he or she is walking, then there is no callback. Patients receive supportive messages, and they do not receive another call until the following week. There is a hierarchical logic used to deliver self-management support. In addition to the telephone intervention, patients attend a weekly surveillance and education session over a 9-month period.

A randomized trial examining usual care provided to diabetic patients and the ATSM intervention was conducted in primary care practices using very broad inclusion criteria (Handley et al., 2008; Sarkar et al., 2008; Schillinger et al., 2009). Schillinger pointed out that usual care at UCSF is fairly robust. In general, patients are seen by a primary care physician, diabetes educators, nutritionists, and when indicated, by specialists (e.g., endocrinologists). When the automated telephone self-management intervention was compared to the adjunctive group medical visits and to usual care in a three-arm comparative effectiveness trial, the level of engagement was much higher for ATSM than for the group medical visits. Engagement was especially high for those with communication barriers of limited literacy or English proficiency. The ATSM group also had the most significant gains in their diabetes self-management behavior at 1 year compared to where they were at a baseline. Quality-of-life outcomes were also enhanced by the automated phone system. For example, days spent in bed sick from diabetes decreased from 3.8 days per month to 1.7 days per month, about a 50 percent reduction in days spent in bed for those who received the automated telephone intervention. The results suggest that this is a promising low-cost technology to redesign the healthcare system and provide an adjunct to care.

The study also demonstrated that the intervention was cost-effective. There has been great interest in the product. Medicaid Managed Care

Plans have expressed interest, with a large majority of Medicaid health plans in California reporting an interest in employing ATSM-like technologies (Goldman et al., 2007). These plans enroll large numbers of diabetics who do not speak English; and if they do, they have limited literacy and numeracy skills. One health plan in San Francisco, with a high number of non-English speaking patients, wanted to adapt and adopt the program for their members with diabetes.

Working with health plans has been very productive. Health plans have skills and resources that are not available in research settings. Their marketing and outreach departments, for example, can identify new enrollees as a Spanish-speaker, Chinese-speaker, or English-speaker, and send an enrollment card for the diabetes program. The program is a covered benefit. The health plan program has been successful in engaging their members with diabetes. On average, 60 percent of the members are picking up and answering these automated calls on a weekly basis. This rate does not appear to diminish over time. The Chinese language speakers are the most engaged, followed by the Spanish speakers, and then the English speakers. This has been a wonderful example of a community-engaged research project, building on a prior RCT.

Another CTSI intervention implemented in both academic and community settings informs and involves people with cancer in their treatment decisions (Jeff Belkora, PI). Breast cancer patients are sent decision aids before their visits (i.e., videos and booklets). During the visit a number of communication aids and techniques are used, including question listing, audio recording, and note taking. After their medical visits, women debrief with a "breast buddy," and decide on a treatment plan. The goal is to integrate evidence-based decision and communication aids into the high-volume academic Breast Care Center at UCSF. The intervention is also being implemented in a rural community setting, Mendocino County, which is about a 4-hour drive north of San Francisco.

Patients reported that the recordings and notes were invaluable in recalling the conversation with the doctor and helpful in clarifying options, understanding the consequences of available choices, and making decisions. Results indicate that the intervention is associated with improved patient knowledge, increased question asking, and improved recall of information. The communication and decision aids have also shifted the time, place, and people who are involved in information exchange. The healthcare experience improved not only for patients, but also for clinicians. Physicians report that the patients coming in with decision aids are more prepared and ask questions that make good use of the available time.

In support of the fourth goal of the National Action Plan to Improve Health Literacy, UCSF, under the leadership of Ricardo Munoz, is attempting to improve linguistically appropriate mental health services by leveraging the Internet and mobile technology. Munoz is director of the Latino Mental Health Research Program at San Francisco General Hospital. He is developing and testing automated self-help Internet interventions and is particularly interested in depression, depression prevention, cognitive behavioral therapy, and recently, smoking cessation. Munoz believes that current health care relies too heavily on consumable interventions. Medications can only be used once. Time spent in a face-to-face intervention can never be used again. In contrast, the Internet can be used more effectively with a greater reach and at marginal cost. The Internet-based smoking-cessation program has been accessed by individuals across the country and internationally. There is a Spanish-language website, and a site is being developed for Chinese speakers. Munoz is tailoring the website content to meet varying levels of literacy.

Schillinger described a multisite heart failure study (Michael Pignone, University of North Carolina, PI, with UCSF, UCLA, and Northwestern University collaborators). In general, one in five Medicare patients who are hospitalized, are hospitalized with heart failure. Investigators compared a single educational session to a tiered educational approach for heart failure patients in reducing heart failure admissions. The inpatient quality measure used by the Center for Medicare and Medicaid Services (CMS) calls for patients to be given written materials regarding such factors as diet, weight monitoring, and medication management. Over 600 patients were enrolled in the trial, including 40 percent who had limited health literacy. The single-session intervention was compared to a goal-directed, layered teaching program using the Teach to Goal approach. The teach-back method is used to ensure that patients understand the core elements of self-management for heart failure, such as the need to weigh oneself daily. Those who were randomized to the Teach to Goal arm had very robust short-term improvements in self-efficacy, heart failure self-care, and heart failure-related quality of life. The gains in quality of life were clinically significant. One-year outcomes look very promising, especially for those with limited health literacy.

Freedman and others have advanced the concept of "public health literacy" (Freedman, 2009). They define it as the degree to which individuals in groups can obtain, process, understand, evaluate, and act upon information needed to make public health decisions that benefit the community. In the case of secondhand smoke, the target population was the public, and the purpose of the educational campaign has been to improve the health of the public. Public health literacy involves engaging stakeholders in public health efforts to address the underlying determinants of health. It also involves many constructs, including some conceptual foundations about the influence of environment on individual health, critical skills, and a civic orientation.

Schillinger pointed out that the public's awareness of the dangers of secondhand smoke is an example of a health literacy success story. The target audience for knowledge about secondhand smoke was the general public. The recognition that one person's smoking behavior is not only bad for that person, but also bad for others in the community was a major accomplishment. According to UCSF researcher Stan Glantz, an estimated 600,000 people a year have been saved as a result of research related to secondhand smoke.

Kirsten Bibbins-Domingo (UCSF Center for Vulnerable Populations, San Francisco General Hospital) studied the overuse of salt and sugar in the diet. It is well established that lowering salt lowers blood pressure. The association between daily salt intake and systolic and diastolic blood pressure is fairly linear. Individuals who consume 8 grams of salt a day have much higher systolic blood pressures than those who take in four, for example. Using a sophisticated modeling technique, Bibbins-Domingo showed that everyone's blood pressure is lowered with lower salt, but the elderly, those who have hypertension, and African-Americans have a greater reduction in blood pressure with lower amounts of salt.

Bibbins-Domingo modeled what would happen to the health of Americans if sodium in processed foods were reduced by 20 to 30 percent, a very modest reduction (Bibbins-Domingo et al., 2010). She found that mortality would fall across all age groups, with the greatest mortality benefit among the young and African Americans. With a reduction in salt intake there would be between a 5 and 12 percent reduction in mortality from cardiovascular disease, stroke, and hypertension. This reduction is equivalent to the public health gains achieved if half of American smokers stopped smoking. This intervention was triple the effect of a 5 percent weight loss among those who were obese. It was 10 times more effective than putting everybody on cholesterol-lowering medications (e.g., statins), and was as effective as having everyone with hypertension on optimal blood pressure treatment.

The World Health Organization estimates it costs a dollar per person to reduce salt through regulatory means, public campaigns, and monitoring. The cost savings are $7 saved for every dollar spent.

Schillinger concluded that salt in foods, and consumption of sugar-sweetened beverages (that is also promoted by high-salt food, which drives the thirst response) are major contributors to the rise in hypertension, diabetes, and obesity in the United States. Public health efforts are needed to change these dangerous trends. Health literacy and interventions and new policies will be key to informing and activating the public to bring about change among individuals, communities, and policy makers, Schillinger said.

WORKFORCE TRAINING AND PREPAREDNESS

Carol Mangione, M.D., M.S.P.H.
University of California, Los Angeles

As mentioned earlier, health literacy is "the degree to which individuals have the capacity to obtain, process, and understand basic health information and services" (Ratzan and Parker, 2000). Only 52 percent of patients understand what health providers tell them or give them to read (IOM, 2004). According to the 2003 National Assessment of Adult Literacy (NAAL), almost 45 percent of the U.S. population (or 93 million Americans) have only basic or below basic literacy skills. The NAAL categorizes "Below Basic" as the ability to perform only the most simple and concrete literacy skills such as signing a form, adding amounts on a bank deposit slip, and searching in a simple text to find out whether a patient is allowed to drink liquids before a medical test.

The NAAL only measures adult literacy, that is, the ability to read. Health literacy is much broader, involving the ability to read, understand, and act upon health information. Numeracy is also an important component of health literacy. The estimates from the NAAL survey are low when the complexity that the health setting confers is taken into consideration.

In 2003 the California Health Literacy Initiative found that 23 percent of California residents lacked basic prose literacy levels. Nearly 70 percent of the immigrants who have resided in California for 10 or fewer years are functionally illiterate. To be functionally illiterate means that you are unable to read the label on a medicine bottle, complete a medical history form, or find an intersection on a street map (http://www.cahealthliteracy.org). Statewide estimates of health literacy are not available, but they are likely to be higher than low literacy levels overall.

Being health literate has become a challenge in light of the increasing complexity of medical care and the healthcare system, Mangione said. Written patient materials that are often lengthy and delivered quickly during stressful medical encounters are being provided to patients to help them understand verbal instructions. Even the most well-educated and experienced individuals can have difficulties navigating the healthcare system.

There is a strong association between low health literacy and processes and outcomes of care. Having low health literacy is associated with delays in diagnosis (Bennet et al., 1998), in poor disease management skills (Williams et al., 1995), and in higher healthcare costs (Weiss et al., 1994).

When physicians were asked, as part of a survey conducted by the California Health Literacy Initiative, whether low literate adults get lower quality of care, 94 percent of physicians said that they thought that was the case (http://www.cahealthliteracy.org). Most (89 percent) physicians, when asked whether they had received any formal training in health literacy, said no. Herein lies the educational challenge, Mangione said.

The survey results identified the need to better understand necessary components of medical professional training and effective methods of instruction. While there are some techniques that are being used by some medical providers, for example, the teach-back method and reduction in the use of medical jargon, Mangione said that more techniques should be tested and applied. The survey results suggest that many physicians have received the message that health literacy, as an issue, exists. This message now needs to be spread to all allied health professionals, including pharmacists, nurses, nurse practitioners, and medical assistants. It is probable that the nursing profession is ahead of physicians on this issue because of their proximity to patients and the amount of time they spend decoding the complex instructions that physicians tend to leave patients with.

There are many challenges when considering the health workforce training needs. First, most of the literature on health literacy has focused on patient factors that put people at greatest risk, whether it is not speaking English as a first language, being an older adult, or not having finished high school. There are relatively few research findings relevant to the workforce of people who care for patients.

When surveyed, health professionals tend to overestimate patients' health literacy. Health professionals do not routinely use many of the best practices for effective communication with patients of low health literacy. The evidence base for understanding whether using these techniques actually improves care is limited to a small number of studies.

The American Medical Association (AMA) Foundation has contributed to understanding educational methods appropriate for health professionals. The AMA has recommended five communication techniques for patients with low literacy (Schwartzberg et al., 2007):

1. Understandable language
2. The teach-back method
3. Patient-friendly materials
4. Helping patients understand
5. Patient-friendly environment

As part of a study of the routine use of communication techniques by physicians, pharmacists, and nurses, investigators from the AMA asked attendees of a health literacy conference about their interactions with patients. Nurses were significantly more likely than physicians and pharmacists to use the teach-back method (60.5 percent, 35.4 percent, and 27.7 percent, respectively). Roughly two-thirds of all the health professionals said that they spoke more slowly, and almost all used simple language and avoided jargon.

The 2004 IOM report *Health Literacy: A Prescription to End Confusion* concluded that "Health professionals and staff have limited education, training, continuing education, and practice opportunities to develop skills for improving health literacy" and recommended that "Professional schools and professional continuing education programs in health and related fields, including medicine, dentistry, pharmacy, social work, anthropology, nursing, public health, and journalism, should incorporate health literacy into their curricula and areas of competence."

The Accreditation Council for Graduate Medical Education (ACGME), the body responsible for the accreditation of post-M.D. medical training programs, has stated that "Residents must demonstrate interpersonal and communication skills that result in the effective exchange of information and collaboration with patients, their families, and health professionals" (ACGME, 2007). Mangione questioned the adequacy of training available to prepare residents to meet this requirement. She also questioned the ability of current medical school faculty to train residents given their own lack of training in this area.

Numerous agencies, including IOM, have called for improvements in training health professionals in health literacy; however, core competencies for health literacy training have not yet been identified. Developing training materials is difficult without first identifying core competencies. Cliff Coleman and colleagues at Oregon Health and Sciences University have a project under way that will define the necessary health literacy–related knowledge, skills, attitudes, and practices for health professionals.

The teach-back technique was identified in 2001 by AHRQ as one of 11 top patient safety practices. This approach asks patients to recall and restate what they have heard during the informed consent process (AHRQ, 2001). The teach-back technique works as part of an interactive communication loop. When a clinician discusses a new concept or provides health information, the clinician assesses the patient's recall and comprehension and clarifies and tailors the information according to what the patient has recalled. According to Mangione, this technique has not been widely taught in California.

There are limited data available for the status of health literacy training, but according to anecdotal reports, health professionals have limited awareness and skills and literacy training is inadequate. Many organizations have recommended that training and curricula be improved, but although curricula is proliferating, and 70 percent of medical schools require some health literacy training, the content and effectiveness of the training are unknown.

Mangione reported on a nonscientific, informal survey of health literacy curriculum for health professionals being trained within the UC system. She sent an e-mail to the five UC School of Medicine deans of education, and the deans of the pharmacy school, two nursing schools, and two schools of public health. She asked for descriptions of their curriculum to prepare health professionals to work with patients with low health literacy. Up to five reminders were sent to encourage response. Replies were received from all but one of her contacts, and the information is displayed in Table 4-1.

Mangione found that when programs had some curriculum content in the area of health literacy the content was often embedded in other coursework and respondents were not able to give precise estimates of the time committed to health literacy or its components. In medical schools, for example, doctoring courses tend to be where doctor-patient communication is taught. The health communication part of the doctoring courses is a logical place to integrate health literacy training.

There is a long tradition of formal training in health communication for physicians, nurses, and pharmacists. However, the structure of this training in health professional schools has traditionally assumed a high

TABLE 4-1 Results of Informal Survey of University of California Health Professional Schools' Health Literacy Curriculum

Campus	Response
UC Berkeley–Public Health	No specific curriculum on health literacy; this topic is included in various courses. Sessions are taught for Joint Medical Program students (Berkeley and UCSF) and for the public health students in Public Health Interventions class as well as in sessions for other professors' courses.
UC Davis–Medicine	Health literacy is embedded in the 3-year Doctoring course.
UC Davis–Nursing	New school—entering class is Masters and Ph.D. level. No specific curricula developed yet.
UC Irvine–Medicine	Through the Reynolds Foundation grant, several sessions in the curriculum touch on health literacy (mainly to address health disparities).
UC Irvine–Nursing	Health literacy is taught throughout the curriculum in both the Adult Health Care course and Community-Based Health Care course for undergraduate nursing students. It is also taught in the Human Behavior and Mental Health courses at the graduate level.

continued

TABLE 4-1 Continued

Campus	Response
UCLA–Medicine	Session held early in the third year curriculum on health literacy. Introduced "teach back" as a technique to verify patient understanding. "Low literacy" guidelines and scenarios developed as teaching resources. Design & Technology unit developing an online module based on presentation by Dr. Fernandez (UCSF).
UCLA–School of Public Health	Many courses in the Community Health Sciences and Health Services Departments describe the prevalence of low health literacy and the implications for communication and care delivery. Additionally, all Masters in Public Health program participants are required to do field work in underserved communities where they witness the impact of low health literacy first hand.
UCSD–Medicine	Included in Clinical Foundations Sequence that all students take during the preclerkship years, and highlighted particularly regarding issues of adherence to therapy and cultural competency.
UCSF–Medicine	Developed interactive presentation on common medical scenarios, possible clinical outcomes, and practical skills for students to use if encountering similar situations. Integrated into online training in health disparities.
UCSF–Pharmacy	Response pending.

SOURCE: Mangione, 2010.

level of both prose and numeric literacy and has not included specific competencies such as teach-back and speaking without using medical jargon. Often, health literacy is incorporated into the part of the curriculum that covers healthcare disparities. While this may be appropriate, Mangione said, such courses may not convey the fact that a large proportion of older adults have very limited health literacy and that it is not a condition that only affects minorities.

There are several unresolved issues in the area of health literacy training, Mangione said. There is little evidence about how much curriculum is enough to achieve competence in communicating with patients who have low health literacy. Preparing patients to succeed in following complex regimens may require a major effort and the use of a variety of tools on the part of providers. Given the high rates of low health literacy in California, health professionals may eventually be required to demonstrate competence in this area, perhaps as a continuing medical education requirement for renewal of a medical license.

One of the most widely known resources for health literacy training for healthcare providers is the AMA Health Literacy Toolkit. The toolkit provides a train-the-trainer type of curriculum. It includes a *Manual for Clinicians*, a video documentary, patient education materials, PowerPoint slides, participant guides, evaluation and reporting forms, and faculty instructions. The course is free online or can be obtained from the AMA bookstore. Over 30,000 physicians and other health professionals have come to training sessions that used the toolkit, and there are 38 healthcare teams that have been trained. Individual training is also available online. The training is free and provides continuing medical education (CME) credit to clinicians who complete it.

In terms of effectiveness, an evaluation of the program has shown changes in clinical practice following the training, Mangione said. Trainees reported a 72 percent increase in asking patients to repeat back instructions, 80 percent reported using simple language and avoiding jargon, and 70 percent reported speaking more slowly after having completed the training. In terms of self-perception, 71 percent reported that they were delivering higher-quality care.

Another training resource is the AHRQ Health Literacy Universal Precautions Toolkit. The universal precautions approach is sensible because it takes a lot of time to judge whether a patient has low health literacy. Practitioners should use good communication approaches no matter who the patient is.

The AHRQ toolkit is designed to help adult and pediatric practices ensure that systems are in place to promote better understanding by all patients. The toolkit is divided into manageable modules so its implementation can fit into the busy day of a practice. It contains a Quick Start Guide, six steps to take to implement the toolkit, 20 different tools, and appendixes with over 25 resources such as sample forms, PowerPoint presentations, and worksheets. Although designed for practices, the toolkit could be integrated into health professional curricula.

The CDC has health literacy online training to educate public health professionals about limited health literacy and their role in addressing it in a public health context. This web-based course can be accessed online. It takes 1.5 to 2 hours to complete (http://www2a.cdc.gov/TCEOnline/registration/detailpage.asp?res_id=2074). Trainees can earn continuing education credits upon course completion. Mangione suggested that the CDC health literacy training program could be used if there were a requirement for licensure related to health literacy training. Medical schools and others could adapt or modify materials that have already been developed.

In addition to these resources that are targeted to continuing education, health literacy curricula have been developed for health professional students at such schools as the University of Chicago, Pritzker School of Medicine.

Health literacy curricula exist for practicing health professionals, and dissemination is under way, Mangione said. Integration of the content of these programs into existing modules on health communication or health disparities in undergraduate curriculum may be the most feasible approach. Reinforcing health literacy knowledge and skills in postdoctoral training also needs to be addressed and the ACGME may have leverage in this area. Consensus on required competencies and assessments are needed. Finally, as is the case for much of medical education, it may be impossible to know how much training is enough. But a stronger focus on health literacy in health professional training and the impact of this training on healthcare quality and safety are needed, Mangione concluded.

DISCUSSION

Roundtable member Bernard Dreyer, in response to Mangione's presentation, discussed the need to teach physicians at multiple levels. At his institution, he said, first-year medical students are taught communication skills, including the teach-back method. He questioned whether the lessons learned at this early stage of training persist until they are needed in practice. Training during residency is very important. There is a free online module on health literacy developed by the American Academy of Pediatrics (available through its online learning center, pedialink.org). Unfortunately, very few residencies have taken advantage of it, Dreyer said, but if the ACGME required it, then every program director would make sure their residents gained this health literacy training.

Dreyer also raised an issue about the universal precautions approach to health literacy. The universal approach is appropriate, but he suggested that very low literacy families or patients really need something more than the universal approach. Perhaps a two-tiered approach is needed.

Dreyer pointed out that the major problem to overcome is changing behavior, and to a lesser extent, knowledge. He and his colleagues conducted a randomized controlled trial in their asthma clinic. All of the physicians used the teach-back method when providing information to patients during the trial. As soon as the trial was over, however, the physicians reverted to their usual behavior. Maintaining good practice is a real issue. More than one-third (37 percent) of the physicians said that they used teach-back consistently. This is likely an overestimate. Dreyer said that a study published in *Pediatrics* showed that 23 percent of practicing pediatricians reported on an anonymous survey that they use the teach-back method with their patients (Turner et al., 2009). Most of them used it occasionally, and not always.

Another issue Dreyer raised is the tendency of clinicians to provide too much information, especially when dealing with a chronic disease. Physicians and nurses both commit this error. With good intentions, they want to give the patient all the available information. However, patients can become overloaded and overwhelmed. It may be advisable to provide two or three messages a visit. Additional messages could be provided on subsequent visits.

Mangione agreed with Dreyer about behavior change. Much of the behavior of physicians is acquired during training through modeling of senior staff and mentors. Reaching more senior clinicians with training on health literacy could improve their ability to serve as appropriate role models. Unfortunately, there are entrenched and engrained poor ways of trying to convey information to patients, and trainees see these poor communication patterns. A sea change is needed in terms of how doctors talk to patients, Mangione said.

Roundtable member Will Ross commented on Schillinger's description of the public health aspects of health literacy. Low health literacy really is a public health threat. Ross asked how to engage more institutions of public health, such as the public health trade associations. Are efforts under way to align these institutions to address population-based health literacy and remove it from the domain of health care? Schillinger referred the question to Rima Rudd, but mentioned that the American Public Health Association (APHA) has been quite engaged in health literacy, and there are a number of public health schools that have been at the forefront in terms of curriculum development. He noted that the crosswalk between schools of public health and schools of medicine, nursing, dentistry, and pharmacy, while helpful when it happens, is not occurring consistently.

Rima Rudd, Harvard School of Public Health, stated that the discipline of public health is far behind in its ability to do research in health literacy, but public health has taken the lead in integrating health literacy into curriculum. The Harvard School of Public Health has offered a course on health literacy since 1992. At Johns Hopkins Bloomberg School of Public Health, health literacy has been taught since the late 1990s. The Society for Public Health Educators (SOPHE), has also taken lead roles in advancing health communication with a focus on health literacy.

Roundtable chair Isham raised the issue of the gap between research and implementation. He found Schillinger's example of the implications to public health of high salt consumption to be a compelling example of the gap between knowledge and remedial action. He suggested that a more active transit system is needed.

5

Improving Health Literacy at the Community Level

NEW YORK CITY MAYOR'S INITIATIVE ON HEALTH LITERACY

Rima Rudd, M.S.P.H., Sc.D.
Harvard School of Public Health

Rudd began her presentation by describing the New York City Health Literacy Initiative as a public health intervention where activities take place outside the healthcare system. Five or 6 years of research, including 3 or 4 years of experimentation and development, preceded the implementation of the initiative. The instruction developed through the initiative was eventually incorporated into the mandated continuing education programs offered statewide for adult educators. The materials for the training of teachers in adult education and the findings from evaluations have been sent to every state department of education in the country. The work has been replicated, adapted, and adopted in multiple states and around the world (e.g., England, Ireland, and Spain).

Within the New York City Mayor's Office of Adult Education, there are three areas focused on health literacy: health literacy and adult education; health literacy fellowships; and the health literacy campaigns Prevention and Detection, Be Active, and Nutrition.

Rudd confined her presentation to the first focus area, health literacy and adult education. The health literacy activities were carried out through a partnership of university collaborators from the Harvard School of Public Health and individuals from a practice agency, the Literacy Assistance Center (LAC) of New York. The LAC focuses on services for adult education teachers, tutors, counselors, job developers, program managers, executive directors, students, researchers, funders, and policy makers. The LAC is the adult education resource for the State of New York and offers student information systems and technical support, a professional development center, a family literacy resource center, and published and online resources.

At the time the health literacy initiatives were being developed in New York, Rudd was a scholar and coinvestigator at the National Center for the Study of Adult Learning and Literacy (NCSALL). The individual scholars and universities comprised by NCSALL were focused on research related to adult learning and literacy. Rudd was the only investigator at NCSALL who conducted research focused on the intersection of health and literacy. Although the level of funding through the U.S. Department of Education was modest, it supported work for 12 years, from 1996 to 2008. The goal for NCSALL was to build and develop research within the adult education field and then translate research into practice.

Throughout her work with NCSALL, Rudd attempted to understand the expectations that health systems had for participating adults and the literacy skills of U.S. adults. She then examined the match (or mismatch) between the expectations and skills. Rudd collaborated with adult education researchers and practitioners, state directors of adult education, teachers and learners, and with representatives of the public health and medical care systems, such as researchers and practitioners in chronic disease specialties, dentistry, mental health, and environmental health. She engaged in a series of studies of health-related activities of adult education programs within states, in programs for adult educators, and in materials and programs for learners to identify the need for collaborative work. Furthermore, Rudd assembled a team of experts across the education and health fields to undergo a "deconstruction" process. This involved an analysis of health-related activities to break down activities (e.g., improving nutrition) into component tasks (e.g., reading food labels, figuring out portion size) and to understand the literacy-related skills people needed to accomplish the tasks as well as to use the tools and materials given to them.

Just before the publication of the 2004 IOM report on health literacy, the New York mayor's office was becoming interested in health literacy and decided to launch a health literacy initiative. The LAC and a number of stakeholders met. At the time, a team with representatives from medicine, nursing, nutrition, adult education, and public health were working to develop a program of study that would enhance the ability of adult educators to develop and teach health literacy skills. With support from NCSALL, the team was developing a series of training manuals for professionals in the adult education sector to help teachers integrate health literacy skills into their programs. The content focus was on three critical issues related to disparities: access to care, managing any chronic disease, and participating in disease prevention and early detection activities. The training manuals were based on a "study circle" process that engages adult educators in collaborative work to examine research findings and then translate those findings into classroom activities.

A pilot site was needed to test the materials. The LAC was eager to pilot the materials and contribute to their development. New York City became the pilot site, and the work became part of the New York City Mayor's Health Literacy Initiative.

Research indicates that people who have limited literacy skills are in triple jeopardy because they have limited access to care, are less likely to participate in screening and disease prevention activities, and are less likely to manage a chronic disease. Consequently, they are seven to eight times more likely to die unnecessarily of a chronic disease. Thus, the focus of the study circles fit well with the population of interest to the LAC and to the City of New York.

Rudd noted that the health literacy study circle activities and materials were not meant to turn adult educators into health educators. Instead, the goal was to focus on the existing expertise of the adult educator and to integrate health-related examples and issues into the classroom with a focus on skills the adult education teacher already teaches. The educators were eager to use health as a context for their teaching because of its relevance to students' lives and to the high interest adult learners have in health-related issues and topics. However, the educators were not particularly interested in teaching health.

The *Study Circle Guidebook* was piloted and improved through this collaborative relationship with the LAC. The LAC staff, experienced in professional development and program implementation, offered in-depth reviews from seasoned experts, venues for facilitator reflections and suggestions, and opportunities to tap into the perceptions and suggestions of participating teachers. The collaboration identified and raised funding for further collaborative work. Three *Health Literacy Study Circle Facilitator Guide* manuals were developed and disseminated.

Financial support for the initiative was inadequate, Rudd said. The director of the LAC was asked to launch the Health Literacy Initiative; however, there was no financial support from the mayor's office. NCSALL resources for the pilot test of their health literacy materials were used for the project. Subsequently, the LAC raised funds for the collaborative work. The LAC and Rudd formed a relationship built on mutual respect and excitement for the undertaking. Rudd turned to the LAC for their literacy expertise, and the LAC turned to Rudd because it knew the interaction would allow the LAC to hone and further develop understanding of adult learners' health literacy as well as teaching techniques, lesson plans, syllabus development, curriculum design, and evaluation methods.

These materials were all developed with a theoretical base in pedagogy and participatory engagement. The processes were based on the pedagogy of Malcolm Knowles and of Paulo Freire. Participants in the study circle engage in an analytic process of discovery, creativity, and group analysis. This process, called Praxis, comes out of Paulo Freire's work. People engage in analysis, gather insights, determine options for putting learning into action, take action, and then come back to the table for reanalysis. The framework for the specific activities within each session was based on Bandura's model of efficacy building and included the facilitator's modeling of possible teaching techniques. Thereafter, the theory of diffusion of innovation was applied to disseminate materials within and throughout the adult education system in every state.

The activities for teachers participating in the study circle mirrored some of the processes undertaken by the initial research team to analyze the expectations for adults' actions related to each area of health disparity. Teachers participating in the study circle identified various health activities and then identified the tasks embedded in an activity as well as the tools needed to accomplish each task. Finally, the teachers identified the literacy skills needed by their students. For example, teachers examined an activity such as taking medicine and were able to identify about 20 different tasks, including going to the pharmacy to obtain the medicine, talking with health professionals, reading and recognizing the name of the medicine, differentiating medicine A from medicine B, reading instructions, and knowing when the medicine goes out of date and needs to be renewed. For every task, they then examined tools needed to accomplish the tasks (e.g., the medicine label), and the literacy skills needed to use each of those tools were identified. Literacy teachers teach reading, speaking and listening skills, as well as numeracy. This deconstruction process was the core of the work and resonated with the teachers.

Teachers participating in the study circle were provided with sample lesson plans (in week 2) that they used or modified in trials with their students. They then developed and tried lesson plans of their own, shared their experiences with fellow participants, and together developed syllabi and evaluation plans. Teachers met for half days, 5 times, with 2 weeks in between. The 2-week break was used to develop lessons and experiment within their classrooms. Study circles are based on the concept of research to practice. Teachers come together, learn about the research that has been done, analyze the relevance of the findings to their own practice, and work together to find ways to apply that research to their practice. The guidebook design is illustrated below (Box 5-1).

Each section of the guidebook includes a booklet that the trainer can

> **BOX 5-1**
> **Guidebook Outline**
>
> - Overview, planning, and facilitation tips
> - Overview and prep for session 1
> - Session 1: Intro to health literacy and [topic]
> - Session 2: Identifying tasks and underlying skills, sample lessons
> - Session 3: Integrating health literacy skills into instruction
> - Session 4: Planning lessons, units, and evaluations
> - Session 5: Developing strategies for success with loose-leaf readings, examples, and handouts
>
> SOURCE: Rudd, 2010.

bring to the training session. It also includes a loose-leaf section with background readings and a comprehensive set of materials that facilitators can replicate for distribution to the participating teachers. Every session is structured the same way. For each session there are notes to facilitators, suggestions for introductory activities, tips on helping participants engage in discussion and analysis, examples of classroom planning tools, closure activities for the session, an evaluation exercise for the session, and an analysis of group discussion methods used in the session that the teachers could then use in their own classrooms. Every training activity was viewed as a modeling opportunity. The facilitator is modeling teaching techniques that the teachers could use in the classroom.

During the first 2 years of the New York City Mayor's Health Literacy Initiative more than 200 teachers were trained, reaching 50,000 adult learners in New York City. An outside group conducted a rigorous first-year evaluation to ensure that programs had shared lessons and expanded expertise, educators built skills, and learners had enhanced skills. In addition, the pilot led to the development of a richer set of materials that were then published. The program and its materials were disseminated through train-the-trainer programs led by the LAC in New York City, in New York State, and then to states around the country. Materials were sent at no cost to every department of education in the country and posted online. The materials have also been used internationally. In addition, relationships were formed within neighborhoods in New York City between adult education programs and local hospitals based on a navigation activity embedded in the access-to-care study circle. One hospital in particular moved ahead to call for community-wide participation in a hospital visit for an introduction to, and overview of, the hospitals' services—an activity that generated wide media coverage. This event also enhanced the reputation of the hospital within the community.

There have been some new more recent developments. For example, partnerships have been formed between health literacy programs and local libraries, hospitals, and hospital groups. In addition, training capacity has been expanded and train-the-trainer programs have taken place in many places throughout the country. Participants of the early study circles went on to facilitate the study circles with other adult education centers.

Partnerships are built on respectful engagements, not through the idea that "I'm going to ask you to do something that I need to have done," but instead, coming together to meet each other's needs and with respect for each partner's area of expertise and with a goal of serving each other's needs. Participatory approaches are needed, Rudd said, so that trainees have the power and the ability to share insights and introduce changes to the process and products. It is important to pay attention to both content and process and to build on the strengths of all partners.

It is important to understand that health literacy is an intersection of skills and demands, Rudd said. Health literacy is not a characteristic of individuals—something that one has, or does not have. Instead, it is composed of skills that can be built. However, while educators can help build these skills, professionals in public health or medicine do not have the capability, the mission, or the time to increase the public's health literacy. Instead, those in health fields need to be attentive to the demand side of the equation. Health providers have a responsibility to remove literacy-related barriers to information and to care. There is ample evidence of the skills of the public. The expectations of healthcare providers must be realistic and activities (e.g., talk, materials, processes) must be in line with people's needs. It is critically important to improve health providers' communication skills.

Rudd's final point focused on the partnership process. The project did not involve one partner in the analytic process and the other in an implementation process. Instead, both partners were engaged in the rigorous development of creative and malleable products and processes that could be replicated, adapted, and adopted.

MiVIA

Cynthia Solomon
FollowMe, Inc.

Solomon began her presentation by describing the motivation behind her involvement in health literacy. As the mother of a child with very complex medical needs (including 18 brain surgeries and 30 hospitalizations) and no easy way to track his care, she began to develop and promote personal health records (PHR), especially for vulnerable populations. Her company's product, MiVIA, is a web-based, patient-owned electronic PHR originally designed for low-income, migrant, agricultural workers. It was well suited to this population as migrants are mobile and when seeking care, access many clinics and health systems. Since its early use in 2003, it has been adapted to meet the needs of anyone with a medical condition, including the homeless, and people with special needs. The tools and resources within the MiVIA PHR help bridge health systems, promote health literacy, facilitate continuity of care, and engage and empower patients to become active care partners, Solomon said. MiVIA ensures security and privacy and is compliant with federal law (i.e., the Health Insurance Portability and Accountability Act [HIPAA] of 1996 [P.L. 104-191]).

The role of the MiVIA PHR is to engage patients by providing them with a place to store and share their medical information. It is also a tool to teach consumers patients' rights, roles and responsibilities, how to interact with the healthcare system, and how to work with providers as a partner in care. The MiVIA PHR helps reduce the digital divide and provides access to health and community services, clinics, libraries, English as Second Language (ESL) programs, and peer-to-peer communications.

One of the keys to the success of MiVIA has been the role of the *promotores de salud*. These Spanish-speaking, community-based, lay workers provide enrollment assistance and training in the use of MiVIA. They also provide cultural and social support, and they check in with clients on their use of MiVIA. There are more than 5,000 MiVIA members in Sonoma County, California.

The training of the *promotores* includes using computers, accessing programs, Internet navigation, and how to enter information into the PHR. The need for privacy and security is highlighted. The training in work groups can be intense, and trainees are encouraged to return for a MiVIA review. The repetition helps the clients gain comfort and confidence.

As of 2010, MiVIA had expanded to six states with 24,000 users. The program serves diverse populations and projects. For example, hospital systems are using MiVIA for their mobile medical units and migrant education. Likewise, county governments use MiVIA for clients that attend their mobile health units. It has provided a low-cost health information exchange system. Community partnerships are being expanded. Solomon pointed out that MiVIA maximizes existing resources.

The addition of audio and video learning tools has enhanced the product. As part of its Effective Healthcare Project, AHRQ developed a series of six 1-minute videos with Ileana Gonzalez, an AHRQ expert who has practiced medicine in her native Nicaragua. Topics include understanding medications, osteoporosis, gestational diabetes, and when to use the emergency department.

Health literacy gains can be realized with the prudent use of computers, the Internet, e-health, and PHRs, said Solomon. For example, colleagues at the University of California, Davis, Department of Adolescent Medicine worked to develop a product similar to MiVIA for homeless adolescents aging out of foster care. Working with teens in a homeless shelter in Sacramento, California, a personal health information system website was developed, www.healthshack.info. The front page of the site is maintained by the youths themselves. The site incorporates a blog, video, mobile texting, and social networking sites such as Facebook and Twitter. These components were necessary for their communication and for training. Solomon described how at the outset of the collaboration, the teens involved would not make eye contact with the MiVIA staff. They did not feel they had a place in this world of importance. However, they were key developers of HealthShack, and today they are youth ambassadors who travel all over the country to educate others.

Another PHR, Follow My Heart, was designed to meet the needs of patients with congenital heart disease. This product was physician inspired and promotes the development of a physician-patient partnership.

Each of the products developed have incorporated what is called granular consent tools. Inside the PHR, the record holder can give permission for certain individuals to access physical health, but not mental health information. Or the record holder could decide to give a mental health provider sole access to sensitive information.

Solomon itemized lessons learned from her 10 years of experience. First, it is important to understand what the consumer needs. Make no assumptions. Second, people do not like to be labeled (example: migrants, homeless, at-risk, vulnerable). Third, it is crucial to build trust through peer-to-peer outreach before deployment. Fourth, it is critical to partner with organizations that speak the same language and share and understand the same culture as the end user. Finally, consumers need to have a sense of ownership and control with assurances of privacy and consent over the use of their health information.

Solomon made several recommendations. It is important, she said to strategically place language-appropriate health information materials in electronic format, including audio and video media. Furthermore, one needs to support and fund health information technology collaborations and inclusion of community-based organizations and agencies that have direct responsibility for underserved populations—it is crucial to have funds at the local level. Solomon recommended that local and state governments promote consumer engagement in health information technology by introducing technology through culturally appropriate efforts and organizations.

PHRs and other consumer tools should be customized to specific populations addressing the cultural issues and providing information using a nonthreatening, nonjudgmental approach, Solomon said. It is important to provide limited (3–5 years) funding for job training for community-based programs such as the *promotores*, health ambassadors, and health advocate programs in doing peer-to-peer outreach and education.

There are, however, numerous barriers, challenges, and realities in the use of health information technology to advance health literacy. There is lack of funding for community-based organizations wanting to adopt innovative health information technology. Another limiting factor is the private sector has no interest in providing support until there is a demonstration of significant revenue streams or opportunities to sell aggregate data. For true system transformation to take place, financial support is needed at the grassroots level, Solomon said.

Having an impact on vulnerable populations in terms of health literacy might require implementing disruptive technologies that serve the consumer, Solomon said. This will promote cost savings to the payer system and redirect funding back to the providers and communities serving these populations.

EMPOWERING PARENTS, BENEFITING CHILDREN, CREATING STRONG FOUNDATIONS FOR HEALTH: IMPROVING HEALTH LITERACY THROUGH THE HEAD START PROGRAM

Ariella Herman, Ph.D., M.S.
University of California, Los Angeles

One million children and families are served every year by Head Start. Services include education and comprehensive health and family services. The program serves families with multiple ethnic, language, and literacy challenges. The Health Care Institute (HCI) at UCLA's Anderson School of Management has had a long-standing relationship with the Head Start program. Twenty years ago, a training program designed for Head Start directors was implemented. To date, the HCI Management Fellows program has trained over 1,200 Head Start directors and managers.

In 2000, Herman surveyed participating Head Start directors about barriers to good health among Head Start participants. Poor health literacy and poor program attendance were identified as obstacles to better health outcomes for families participating in Head Start (Herman, 2000).

> **BOX 5-2**
> **Goals of the HCI Health Literacy Program**
>
> 1. Provide a strategic model for agencies serving families and their young children to successfully implement health literacy education programs.
> 2. Build a better future for vulnerable children by providing their parents with skills and knowledge to
>   a. enable them to become better caregivers by improving healthcare knowledge and skills,
>   b. empower them in health decision making, and
>   c. enhance their self-esteem and confidence in dealing with health issues.
>
> SOURCE: Herman, 2010.

In response to these findings, HCI identified health literacy within Head Start as its primary research focus. Its mission is to help agencies work with young children and their families to provide culturally sensitive, low literacy, health education programs. The goals of the HCI health literacy program are in Box 5-2.

In 2001, Herman engaged with Head Start agencies and planned a health literacy intervention. The key tool that emerged is the Health Improvement Project, shown in Figures 5-1 and 5-2. The first step of the project involves training the trainer, in this case Head Start staff. Teams from Head Start agencies experience 2 days of instruction from faculty from the Anderson School of Management. The training provides staff with skills to effectively market their program within their agency, to their families, and to their communities. The topic of motivation, both staff motivation and parent motivation, is emphasized. Mock training sessions are held where trainees role-play being Head Start parents. Over time, the project also brought in Head Start directors that had been through the program to share with new trainees examples of successes and failures.

Following training, each agency team goes back to their local setting and begins to implement the plan for training. A few months later, the parents whose children attend Head Start participate in a 3-hour training session. Participation has been very good; nationally, about 85 percent of parents attend the session. After the parent training, three home visits are made. This contact with the families helps reinforce both the messages from the training and positive behavioral changes. A graduation ceremony acknowledges parent participation in the training. Data are collected to monitor program effectiveness, including self-assessments of knowledge and behavior, and tracking of health behaviors and outcomes

IMPROVING HEALTH LITERACY AT THE COMMUNITY LEVEL

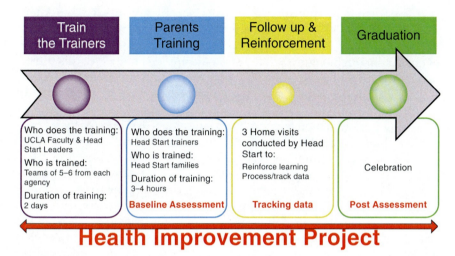

FIGURE 5-1 HCI health improvement project.
SOURCE: Herman, 2010.

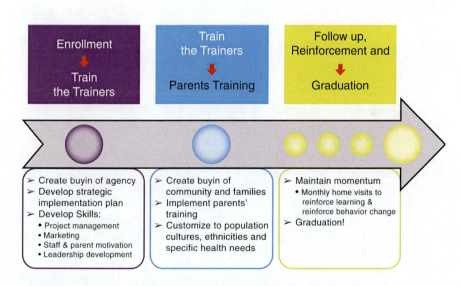

FIGURE 5-2 HCI strategic implementation.
SOURCE: Hermann, 2010.

(e.g., emergency room visits, clinic visits, school days missed, workdays missed) (Figure 5-1). The entire program rolls out in alignment with the school year, from the beginning of planning to the final graduation event. As shown in Figure 5-2, the strategic implementation of this project occurs in three phases: from the enrollment until the train-the-trainer; from the train-the-trainer until the parent training; from the follow-up until the graduation.

An important lesson learned, Herman said, is the need for the agency to create buy-in from Head Start staff, realizing that staff are overworked. A strategic implementation plan is needed to identify how the Head Start agency will accomplish its goals. For example, how will the agency approach the community to get in-kind support? Bringing the community to the training is one way to inspire the community. An example of community engagement is bringing medical residents from a local hospital to participate in the training so they interact with their patients and develop a relationship.

To motivate a poor family to come for parent training one must remove all the barriers, which means providing transportation, childcare, a meal, and creating excitement. To create excitement for parents and motivate their involvement, Head Start staff has to feel excited about the program.

Another lesson learned from collaboration with the Head Start agencies is that the program must be customized. For example, one cannot simply translate materials from one language to another and expect the program to be equally effective in the other language. To reach a particular ethnic group, any program needs to be adapted to that group's specific language and cultural needs. Herman described how one parent training event was conducted in seven languages simultaneously.

A final ingredient of success, Herman said, is keeping the community engaged to maintain momentum, year after year. One might call this ingredient the L.O.V.E. principle: Listening, Observing, Valuing, and Encouraging. This principle is applied to all levels of the program—the management team, the Head Start staff, the teachers, and the parents. The logic model used is to involve staff, children, and parents in the program in order to have an impact on knowledge, behavior, and sustainability.

Herman described some of the outcomes of the Head Start health literacy program. Before the intervention, when asked, "When your child is sick, where do you first go for help?" more than two-thirds (68.9 percent) of parent participants replied that they would seek help from a doctor. Following the intervention, the percentage of parents reporting a doctor as the first source of help declined to 32.6 percent (Table 5-1). The intervention prompted participants to increasingly rely first on printed low-literacy health materials for help.

TABLE 5-1 Parents' Sources of Help When a Child Is Sick

Source	Preintervention (%)	Postintervention (%)
Book	4.7	47.6
Doctor	68.9	32.6
Emergency room	4.4	0

SOURCE: Herman and Mayer, 2004.

The increased reliance on books and on skills learned in the sessions reduced unneeded utilization of healthcare resources. There was a 42 percent decline in number of doctor visits, a 29 percent decline in school days missed, and a 42 percent decline in workdays missed when these events were tracked over the first 8 years of the program. Emergency room visits also declined (Herman and Mayer, 2004).

Based on these changes in healthcare service use, a conservative calculation of cost savings was computed. Assuming $80 for a doctor visit and $320 for an emergency visit, there is $554 savings in healthcare costs per family trained per year. The average cost of this program is $100. This estimate did not take into consideration many other qualitative outcomes and benefits of the program. The program and, in particular, the use of the health reference book led to an increase in parental awareness of health warning signs, a better understanding of common childhood illnesses, and quicker responses to early signs of illness. Parents were also empowered to appropriately use the healthcare system. Figure 5-3 presents an overview of the program's model, impacts, and outcomes.

Research is linked to practice in two ways, Herman said. The first linkage is through effective implementation that involves building capacity, developing leadership, providing tools for strategic project management and replication, and enhancing community outreach. The second linkage is through health promotion that involves using materials that are culturally sensitive and understandable, offering a portfolio of health topics, teaching health skills, and addressing health decision making. Modules have been developed on common childhood illness, oral health, obesity, prenatal education, and how to read over-the-counter medication labels.

The program has trained 45,000 families, 1,150 trainers, and 189 agencies in 45 states, in seven languages, and has adapted the program for successful implementation in 10 ethnic groups. This year, the program moved beyond Head Start and has provided programs within two school districts. The program has corporate and public financial support.

There is one module that addresses obesity and diabetes prevention. This module educates staff, parents, *and* children. The program has succeeded in improving children's nutrition knowledge, eating behavior,

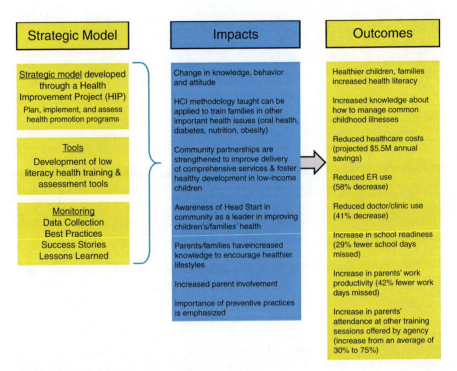

FIGURE 5-3 Overview of the Head Start intervention.
SOURCE: Herman, 2010.

physical activity, and body mass index (BMI). Children were taken to a farmers market and then that experience was used to teach math and science. Parents' BMI improved also, and there was a link between the BMI change of the children relative to the parents. This example illustrates how such a trilevel early intervention can prompt changes within a whole community.

Herman expressed her desire to reach the entire Head Start community. Focusing on prevention and early education is critical, she said. Parents can become the strongest advocates for children if they are given appropriate tools. To be effective, programs must be designed to understand local needs and to motivate members of the community. Entire communities must be engaged. HCI has learned that what is communicated and how communication occurs matters. Appropriate tools need to be provided in a respectful and culturally sensitive way. Parents need to be allowed to assume the primary role of decision making in the care of their children.

Herman concluded by summarizing HCI's vision. That vision is to

- expand reach to all vulnerable families to help reduce health literacy in the nation;
- approach the problem from a population perspective with scalable programs;
- focus on prevention;
- recognize parents are key to advocating for the health and well-being of their families;
- empower families with knowledge, tools, resources, and self-efficacy/self-confidence so they can actively participate in health decisions;
- engage families to achieve sustainable adoption of healthy lifestyle choices; and
- work with communities to develop social capital.

Empowered families can make a difference, Herman said. They can change communities, and they will lead to a healthier nation.

HEALTH LITERACY AT THE UNIVERSITY OF CALIFORNIA, SAN DIEGO, STUDENT-RUN FREE CLINIC PROJECT AND FELLOWSHIP IN UNDERSERVED HEALTH CARE: LEARNINGS

Ellen Beck, M.D.
University of California, San Diego

Beck recounted a lesson learned early in her career while directing a health education program for the elderly. She had been somewhat discouraged in trying to teach medical students how to consistently take a medical history, so she decided she would teach elderly patients how to give a medical history. This was a success, and the patients reported how much they enjoyed walking into the doctor's office and speaking to their doctor using what they had learned, "I told him my chief complaint, and then I went on to my history of present illness, and then I gave him my past medical history." This is just one example of the potential benefits of teaching patients to learn to speak in their doctor's language.

The Student-Run Free Clinic Project (SRFCP), founded in 1997 by a group of University of California, San Diego (UCSD) medical students, outstanding community partners, and Beck, engage in health literacy-related work. The project serves a variety of diverse patients and partners. For example, an older African-American couple who marched with Martin Luther King from Selma to Montgomery helped start one of the free clinic sites, at Baker Elementary School, that serves the surrounding community. A Hispanic member of the community, and former patient of the clinic, first volunteered and is now employed as the project's lead health promoter (*promotora*). A formerly homeless man has become one of the project's street homeless health promoters.

There are now four sites. Two are located in churches that have a long-standing history of providing services to the underserved. Two other sites are located in inner-city elementary schools.

The free clinic project can be considered a safety net for the safety net. San Diego has very limited health services for the poor and uninsured, and many individuals fall through the cracks. For example, a U.S. citizen living in San Diego, who cannot afford health insurance, and thus is in need of county health services must earn less than $1,490 a month to receive such services. In addition, the individual must have a disease that might lead to serious complications, disability, or death. Finally, the person has to sign a lien against any future property to cover healthcare expenditures.

The SRFCP provides continuous, comprehensive, high-quality, outpatient health care to 2,000 people who are without access to care. If a prospective client is eligible for insurance or healthcare elsewhere, such as at a community health center, the SRFCP helps the individual access those services. The SRFCP serves a demographically and socially diverse population, 51 percent Latino, 30 percent Caucasian, and 25 percent street homeless. Most patients (over 85 percent) have at least one serious chronic illness, most commonly, hypertension, diabetes, hyperlipidemia, asthma, or depression.

The clinic has adopted a core philosophy that is taught, modeled, and expected throughout all activities. The components of this philosophy are patient empowerment, humanistic care, transdisciplinary care, and an understanding that the community is the teacher. Trainees are also taught the behaviors associated with these key principles and are evaluated in terms of their adherence to these principles. The SRFCP provides training for students of medicine, pharmacy, acupuncture, dentistry, social work, and law.

Empowerment means creating an environment in which a person can take charge of his or her life and achieve health and well-being. The clinic sponsors a Spanish language empowerment group (formerly called a support group). Beck shared a few personal experiences from the groups. One patient who had been a member of the group for 3 years said,

> When I first came to the group, I was carrying a lot on my shoulders, and I let everything out. I cried a lot. And since then, everybody in the group has helped me to think, to defend myself, to move forward without fear. Everything I hear here I share with my family, and they also are changing. I was in the hospital recently, and they gave me a lot of support. I want this group to continue and want to invite a lot of people so they can listen and learn not to have fear and to move forward. This is my home, and I want to share it with everybody.

Another patient who had been a member of the empowerment group for 4 years said,

> Before coming to this group, I did not know how to control my temper, and I did not know how to speak with my children or my husband. Now I feel like a different person. I know how to control my temper. I know how to speak to my children. Now I know how to get along with myself better. Before, I didn't value myself. I didn't take time for myself. I feel much better about myself. Thanks to all of you. For me, this group is like a family, something beautiful that happened in my life, this experience, this support . . . Ojalá! I wish I can continue to come and to share.

Many of the SRFCP's patients have become volunteers, and they help with the day-to-day clinic functioning. There is a rule that if you attend an empowerment group, it must be as a member and not in the role of a volunteer or professional. The groups are usually conducted in Spanish.

The underlying philosophy of the clinic is humanistic, based on work by Carl Rogers, the founder of humanistic psychology, and the person who coined the phrases, "client-centered," "person-centered," and "patient-centered." Rogers said that the essential qualities of all successful encounters, and especially the therapeutic encounter, required the three elements of empathy, congruence, and respect (Zimring, 1994). Thus, the students are taught and the faculty models that in every client encounter, the SRFCP providers are expected to demonstrate empathy, respect, and congruence. Empathy is a sense of what the patient might be feeling; respect is shown to all in all contexts. Students are taught that they may not respect what a person has done, but they can still show respect to the person as a human being, and that all human beings deserve to be treated with respect. Congruence is self-awareness on the part of the provider, an awareness of what is being experienced and felt in the moment and how that awareness affects the patient encounter. One of the clinic's goals is to dispel hierarchies, stereotypes, and interprofessional prejudices. The clinic philosophy is taught through examples, role modeling, weekly reflection sessions, community building, writing, and didactic sessions that cover topics such as health promotion, health education, working with interpreters, and social resources.

Of the 122 medical students in the first year class at UCSD, 105 students choose to take an intensive elective in order to work at the SRFCP. Throughout first and second year, there are another 70 students who continue to work at the SRFCP as they learn to take on administrative and clinical roles under the supervision of faculty. Some students participate in the clinic during their third year, and 80 fourth-year students elect one of two 4-week clerkships, one in family medicine, and one in undeserved medicine, both of which include intensive experience in the SRFCP. Many of the fourth-year students will be pursuing specialty residencies, for example, radiology, pathology, and anesthesiology, and yet they elect to gain experience at the free clinic. The clinic also offers training to students of pharmacy, dentistry, acupuncture, social work, and law.

Students rotating through the free clinic project learn to teach. Incorporating health literacy into clinical practice requires teaching skills. Fellows in Underserved Health Care teach the fourth-year medical students, and the fourth-year medical students learn to coach first-year students. The senior and junior students see patients together under the supervision of primary care clinicians, most of whom have extensive experience at the SRFCP. An adult health education model is used to teach the medical students how to incorporate health education and health promotion into their practice.

Beck attributed the positive medical outcomes (Table 5-2) of 182 diabetic patients seen at the free clinic and then assessed after receiving care at the free clinic for 1 year to the sense of community, the trust of the patients, the time taken by the students to interact with the patients, and the overall philosophy of care. Students are instrumental in helping patients take charge of their health.

Another program started through the free clinic is a comprehensive wellness program at an inner-city elementary school, Golden Avenue Elementary in the Lemon Grove School District. The program addresses the needs of children, teachers, parents, and the environment. The intervention involves providing access to care for the parents. There are community gardens and a mural program, which involves the community

TABLE 5-2 Outcomes of 182 Diabetic Patients Seen at the UCSD Free Clinic and Assessed at 1 Year

Test	Test Completed Within the Last Year (%)	Percent with Test Result
Blood pressure	100	46% < 130/80 77% < 140/90
Hemoglobin A1C	99	Mean HA1C value = 8.26%
Low-density lipoprotein (LDL)	93	70% < 100 86% < 130
Triglyceride (TG)	88	—
High-density lipoprotein (HDL)	88	—
Microalbumin	80	—

SOURCE: Marrone et al., 2010.

and improves the environment. For teachers, the focus of the intervention is professional renewal. There is a wellness curriculum for the children that involves creative expression (e.g., art, dance, and theater) as well as nutrition and exercise. In addition, the children themselves increase their health literacy and act as health literacy advocates by becoming junior health promoters and participating in an after school prehealth profession program called, "Blue Band-Aid" brigade. The classes provide activities to increase the children's knowledge and skills related to common health issues.

Several health literacy and empowerment methods are used at the SRFCP, Beck said. When clinic providers use the teach-back method, they do not simply ask the patient to repeat information that the provider has discussed. They often ask the patient to pretend that he or she is the doctor and to teach the provider what the provider just taught them. Free clinic providers also learn to ask patients about barriers that may be preventing them from taking charge of their lives and their health. Providers then work with the patient to reduce those barriers. Trainees learn to write personal prescriptions for patients about their sources of strength to overcome barriers. Providers also learn to work with their clients to address client concerns about using fear management tools. During their encounters with patients, providers consider social determinants of health, such as income and social environments. These activities, in addition to learning to build trust, address stigma, and improve knowledge, are all essential ingredients of health literacy training. Beck emphasized the importance of not only working with clients on their health literacy, but also acting to improve clinician health literacy.

Community health workers who interact primarily with the Hispanic community, called *promotores*, come to the medical school to teach students. They are introduced as wise community members, health promoters who have a role at the free clinic, especially in developing and maintaining community trust and partnership. The *promotores* are available during clinic hours to help problem solve and consult. They also cofacilitate the clinic's empowerment group. The free clinic's community partners (e.g., hosts at each site, social workers) are involved in the weekly reflection sessions at the SRFCP.

Student-perceived self-efficacy relates to caring for traditionally underserved patients. Self-efficacy improved dramatically as measured before and after the students' first free clinic elective.[1] Students also reported an increased interest in primary care and increased interest in

---

[1] Beck said this finding comes from an independent study project involving 431 medical students who took the free clinic elective in 2001.

working with underserved populations following their exposure to the clinic.

A 1- to 2-year UCSD Fellowship in Underserved Health Care has enrolled six medical fellows, two dental fellows, and one acupuncture fellow. This fellowship occurs after residency training and is for health professionals interested in devoting their career to underserved health care. The fellows help direct the free clinic and complete a research project and training. Of these fellows, eight of nine were student free clinic leaders who returned after residency to help run the free clinic project. All now devote their careers to working with the underserved.

Beck has also worked to develop a national faculty training program entitled Addressing the Health Needs of the Underserved. Since 1999 this program has enrolled 135 faculty from 30 states. One-quarter of them are from underrepresented minorities in the health professions. The three areas of focus of the training program are faculty development skills, community partnerships and programs, and personal and professional renewal. Overall confidence of trainees in essential knowledge relevant to care of underserved populations increased markedly when measured before and after the training program. For example, improvements were noted in student confidence about creating student curricula related to underserved communities, designing a student- or resident-run free clinic, and developing an educational component or experience that addressed issues of culture and race (Beck et al., 2008). An outcomes study performed after the first 53 participants of the program had completed the program demonstrated that participants had started many student-run free clinics, developed curricula, written their first grants, and assumed new leadership roles.

Beck outlined key lessons learned from her experiences. She emphasized the importance of a sense of ownership by all participants in the SRFCP and other training programs that she has been involved with. The medical students succeed at this work when they have a sense of ownership and when the health literacy work is relevant to their ability to perceive themselves as a future good doctor. If the patient has a sense of ownership and the student has ownership, things work. Beck indicated that in her experience, role modeling and coaching are among the most effective teaching tools. Students need to be taught to be teachers. They also need to learn that patients and the community are truly the teachers. Community member involvement is essential in all aspects of training, teaching, and role modeling. Students need to be oriented to this type of humanistic, empowering transdisciplinary philosophy and to have specific expectations for performance made clear to them.

Lack of health literacy is an injustice, Beck said. As Martin Luther King said, "Injustice anywhere is a threat to justice everywhere." She encouraged the group to continue to address this injustice and, together, to discover creative ways to intervene and change the status quo.

DISCUSSION

Roundtable member, Will Ross, remarked on the success of the interventions described during the workshop and pointed out that some of the success can be traced to the fact that the interventions are based on good public health theory. He pointed out that the theories of diffusion of innovation, community-based planning, and constructs from social cognitive theory are not normally taught in health professional schools. These constructs have been well interwoven into the interventions described during the workshop. Ross mentioned the difficulty of taking a large issue like health literacy and implementing interventions to improve it within the community. In his view health literacy needs to be better integrated into health professional curriculums so core skills are acquired related to behavioral health theory and community planning.

Rudd responded and reiterated the importance of a theory-based approach to health literacy. Of critical importance also is the need for respect for clients and partners, she said. Adult learners, parents, farm workers, and others who might attend health literacy programs need to be treated with a level of respect and dignity so they recognize themselves as empowered agents, and not as subjects.

Beck added that from a medical school education perspective, students should be taught behavioral and social sciences once they have been directly involved in clinical care. Ideally the teaching is concurrent with these clinical experiences. Otherwise, the material is not perceived as relevant. These disciplines become more relevant after the student has had experiences, such as the death of a patient, or being in the emergency room and unable to communicate with a family. Students often learn best when they encounter cases that are challenging and when they are not sure of the best approach or how to cope with their reactions.

Conrad Person, Johnson & Johnson, asked the panel what companies that manufacture health products should be considering making their products more accessible to people. He pointed out that many resources are expended to develop materials that are meant to facilitate the use of products and enhance their effectiveness. These materials, however, do not always meet the needs of people with poor health literacy.

Solomon responded that companies could help sponsor health literacy projects that would lead to video and audio tools on some of the e-learning applications, both for electronic medical records and personal health records. In addition, companies could sponsor some educational programs in the area of medication management. Assisting people with financial support so they could take advantage of some of these tools would also be very helpful, especially in the e-learning arena.

Roundtable chair Isham observed that some advantaged segments of the population tend to overuse commercial products and disadvantaged populations underuse certain products. Companies such as Johnson & Johnson are particularly rich in skills and talents in terms of market segmentation and being able to target particular audiences. There is tremendous social purpose that can be aligned with their economic objectives in terms of more carefully trying to address these disparities. The challenge is to make that alignment work both for the private companies as well as those populations.

Beck added that ideally, a product could be designed like some of the newer thermometers. A button on the packaging could be pushed and instructions in either English or Spanish could be selected and provide information in simple terms on how to use the product. As more people are learning how to navigate the Internet, instructions could be made available online. Solomon suggested a technological intervention that might be helpful: having patients able to pass the bar code on a product over a small machine that would either provide voice instruction or print out instructions in the language of choice.

Jan French, Los Angeles Best Babies Network, leads healthcare improvement collaboratives focused on prenatal and postpartum care in Los Angeles [LA] County. She asked Herman about leveraging resources within communities and at the state and national levels. French mentioned a local resource, the First 5 LA program,[2] and on the federal level, she noted the Promise Neighborhoods Initiative of the Department of Education[3] and the Patient Protection and Affordable Care Act expansion of home visitation programs to disseminate programs that work.[4] Herman responded by describing programs that the HCI is involved with in LA

---

[2]This organization was created by California voters to invest tobacco tax revenues in programs to improve the lives of children in LA County, from prenatal care through interventions for children up to age 5 (http://www.first5la.org/, accessed February 16, 2011).

[3]Promise Neighborhoods provides grant funding to support nonprofit organizations and institutions of higher education to significantly improve the educational and developmental outcomes of children in distressed communities, including rural and tribal communities (http://www2.ed.gov/programs/promiseneighborhoods/index.html, accessed February 16, 2011).

[4]The act provides funding for the Maternal, Infant, and Early Childhood Home Visiting Program. The program relies on evidence-based home-visiting strategies that help families create a nurturing environment for young children and connect to a range of services, including health, early education, and early intervention. The Health Resources and Services Administration (HRSA) administers the program in collaboration with the Administration for Children and Families (ACF) (http://www.hrsa.gov/about/news/pressreleases/2010/100610.html, accessed February 16, 2011).

County. HCI has worked with five Early Head Start programs, seven Head Start programs, and two school districts in LA County. In terms of leveraging, Herman mentioned the importance of emphasizing community partnerships in training programs.

Shannon Alvarado of Lenox School district in LA County discussed her work with Herman. Following a train-the-trainer session in 2010, 120 parents in the school district attended an education program. The Lennox School district occupies a 1.3 square mile area near the L. airport. Most of the children in the district qualify for free or reduced lunches. The parents have used the course materials. A second cycle of parent training took place in early 2011. The work within the school district was highlighted in an article published in the *Los Angeles Times* in October 2010.[5] Ms. Alvarado described the excitement of parents as they learned how to take charge of their children's health.

---

[5]See http://articles.latimes.com/2010/oct/20/local/la-me-head-start-20101020, accessed February 16, 2011.

6

Closing Remarks

Roundtable chair Isham invited members of the roundtable to reflect on the day's proceedings. Roundtable member Benard Dreyer reflected on the relevance of the adage, "all politics is local," to health literacy and suggested that health literacy is also effectively implemented at the local level. He was extremely impressed with the accomplishments and success of the state-level coalitions and suggested that health literacy coalitions be broadly disseminated so they are present in every state. State-based health literacy coalitions are filling a vacuum that exists because state governments, health departments, and agencies that should be focusing on health literacy are not currently engaged. Furthermore, if the state coalitions ceased to exist, there would not be a statewide infrastructure to maintain health literacy activities, he said. There is a need, he said, to motivate the state agencies to incorporate health literacy efforts.

In reflecting on the workshop presentations addressing medical education, Dreyer stated there is much to be done to reach medical students, residents, and faculty members. He indicated progress likely could be made through organizations such as the Association of American Medical Colleges (AAMC) that focus on curriculum, and the Liaison Committee on Medical Education (LCME) and the Accreditation Council for Graduate Medical Education (ACGME) that address regulatory issues. Essential to improving the ability of clinicians to effectively communicate with patients are the experiences available to them while in training. He indicated the experiences medical students and other trainees have in Beck's UCSD free clinic program can be life changing. Medical schools and other clinical training programs need to make these sorts of opportunities available.

Finally, Dreyer said, changes are needed in the health system in order to improve health literacy because focusing on these systematic changes is more important than a misguided attempt at labeling the patient and trying to implement change at that level. But the workshop also affirmed the need to effectively help patients by empowering them to be able to take responsibility for their health care and to ask questions and interact in an empowered way with the healthcare system. Dreyer said the most effective way to improve patient knowledge is by reaching him or her through community outreach and not via the healthcare system. Health providers must work with community partners in a transdisciplinary fashion to achieve success.

Culbert mentioned that the work of Health Literacy Missouri takes place both inside and outside the healthcare system. He cited the importance of focusing on the individual, not in a way that points the finger at them, but rather one that empowers them. It is very important to begin early with individuals, whether they are new mothers, children, or medical students. Reinforcement must take place continuously throughout the life cycle. The state of health literacy will likely take a generation to make advances. Culbert said that progress can be made if there is a commitment to health literacy and efforts are based on good evidence. Knowledge is improving regarding what works at the community level and how to empower individuals so they can make good health decisions.

Roundtable member Winston Wong discussed the implementation of the Patient Protection and Affordable Care Act (ACA) and how health literacy may or may not be a mitigating factor toward the success of its implementation. The ACA will have its impact at the local level. Patient empowerment takes place both in clinicians' rooms and in the community, such as within Head Start programs. There is a need to identify competencies of providers in terms of their ability to empower patients. More functional healthcare encounters would take place if patients were assertive and comfortable specifying their needs and expecting to be heard.

Wong mentioned that 90 percent of Americans do not see a physician or a nurse in any given year, and so much of the effort toward improving health literacy must be directed toward population management and wellness prevention efforts. Health literacy is a key element of how communities try to optimize health and wellness, aside from what happens during a clinical visit. There needs to be a focus on how health literacy is operationalized in terms of changing the trajectory of chronic disease and prospects for wellness and health in communities.

Roundtable member Cindy Brach mentioned that patient empowerment and self-management are focus areas of the AHRQ Health Literacy

Universal Precautions Toolkit. Patient empowerment can be thought of in terms of patients being able to take charge of their own health as opposed to taking charge of the encounter. Fostering patient empowerment is critical to achieving success, Brach said, because it is such a determinant of patient behavior beyond the clinical encounter.

In terms of provider education, Brach mentioned that a number of states have begun to require cultural competency training for licensure. She indicated that a study of the impact of these compulsory training requirements is needed. There are concerns that poor or ill-timed training may not have the results that are desired. Roundtable member Leonard Epstein mentioned the possibility of a collaborative study of these state requirements that would involve the Health Resources and Services Administration (HRSA).

Epstein stated that he was going to take several of the lessons he gleaned from the workshop back to HRSA's various offices and bureaus that address the education and training of health professionals, the needs of mothers and children, and the provision of care in community health centers. There are potential implementation and research projects that could be initiated to further the work of the presenters. Mr. Epstein referred to a favorite saying of one of the early directors of the Bureau of Primary Healthcare, Marilyn Gaston, "Good primary health care is done community by community."

Isham highlighted the importance of a national system of standards, discipline, and attention to health literacy at different levels of jurisdiction, national and state, in terms of health reform, and most importantly at the community level, where implementation occurs. It is not a matter of one versus the other, but the right mix of national, state, and community efforts. A major challenge is dissemination, that is, consistently applying model programs across the country.

Isham indicated that the workshop sessions provided examples of disseminating research findings from academia to clinical practices and community settings. There were also examples of incorporating research into clinical practices and offering clinical training in the community. The workshop included descriptions of innovative programs from North Carolina, Iowa, Missouri, and Louisiana that serve as models for other states to emulate. These types of integrative efforts are needed, Isham said. Challenges remain in terms of breaking down barriers between research institutions, clinical practices, and communities.

Isham also emphasized the need for theory-based interventions and for disciplined thinking. There are tremendous opportunities for a different kind of partnership between academics and practically minded people in the community. He also emphasized the importance of health literacy in addressing healthcare quality.

Isham concluded the workshop by expressing thanks for the fruitful collaboration between the UCLA Anderson School of Management and the roundtable.

References

Abrams, M.A. 2010. *The Iowa experience: Creating a shared vision for health literacy in Iowa.* Presented at the Institute of Medicine workshop on Understanding What Works in Improving Health Literacy Within a State, November 30, 2010.

Accreditation Council for Graduate Medical Education (ACGME). 2007. *Common program requirements: General competencies approved by the ACGME board February 13, 2007.* http://www.acgme.org/outcome/comp/GeneralCompetenciesStandards21307.pdf (accessed February 10, 2011).

AHRQ (Agency for Healthcare Research and Quality). 2001. *Making health care safer: A critical analysis of patient safety practices.* Summary (Publication No. 01-E057); Evidence Report (Publication No. 01-E058). University of California, San Francisco: Evidence-Based Practice Center. http://archive.ahrq.gov/clinic/ptsafety/summary.htm.

AHRQ. 2010. *Health literacy universal precautions toolkit.* AHRQ Publication No. 10-0046-EF. Rockville, MD: AHRQ. http://www.ahrq.gov/qual/literacy/index.html.

Beck, E., D. L. Wingard, M. L. Zúñiga, R. Heifetz, and S. Gilbreath. 2008. Addressing the health needs of the underserved: A national faculty development program. *Academic Medicine* 83(11):1094-1102.

Bennett, C. L., M. R. Ferreira, T. C Davis, J. Kaplan, M. Weinberger, T. Kuzel, M. A. Seday, and O. Sartor. 1998. Relation between literacy, race, and stage of presentation among low-income patients with prostate cancer. *Journal of Clinical Oncology* 16(9):3101-3104.

Bibbins-Domingo, K., G. M. Chertow, P. G. Coxson, A. Moran, J. M. Lightwood, M. J. Pletcher, and L. Goldman. 2010. Projected effect of dietary salt reductions on future cardiovascular disease. *New England Journal of Medicine* 362(7):590-599.

Freedman, D. A., K. D. Bess, H. A. Tucker, D. L. Boyd, A. M. Tuchman, and K. A. Wallston. 2009. Public health literacy defined. *American Journal of Preventive Medicine* 36(5):446-451.

Goldman, L. E., M. Handley, T. G. Rundall, and D. Schillinger. 2007. Current and future directions in Medi-Cal chronic disease care management: A view from the top. *American Journal of Managed Care* 13(5):263-268.

Handley, M. A., M. Shumway, and D. Schillinger. 2008. Cost-effectiveness of automated telephone self-management support with nurse care management among patients with diabetes. *Annals of Family Medicine* 6(6):512-518.

Herman, A. 2000. *The status of health care in Head Start: A descriptive study*. Los Angeles, CA: UCLA Anderson School of Management.

Herman, A. 2010. *Empowering parents, benefiting children, creating strong foundations for health: Improving health literacy through the Head Start program*. Presentation at the Institute of Medicine workshop on Understanding What Works in Improving Health Literacy Within a State, November 30, 2010.

Herman, A. D., and G. G. Mayer. 2004. Reducing the use of emergency medical resources among Head Start families: A pilot study. *Journal of Community Health* 29(3):197-208.

HHS (U.S. Department of Health and Human Services). 2010. *National action plan to improve health literacy*. Washington, DC: Department of Health and Human Services, Office of Disease Prevention and Health Promotion.

Hickson, G. B., and A. D. Jenkins. 2007. Identifying and addressing communication failures as a means of reducing unnecessary malpractice claims. *North Carolina Medical Journal* 68(5):362-364. http://www.ncmedicaljournal.com/wp-content/uploads/NCMJ/sep-oct-07/hickson.pdf.

IOM (Institute of Medicine). 2001. *Crossing the quality chasm: A new health system for the 21st century*. Washington, DC: National Academy Press.

IOM. 2004. *Health literacy: A prescription to end confusion*. Washington, DC: The National Academies Press.

The Joint Commission. 2007. *"What did the doctor say?": Improving health literacy to protect patient safety*. Oakbrook Terrace, IL: The Joint Commission.

The Joint Commission. 2008. *Strategies for improving health literacy*. The Joint Commission Perspectives on Patient Safety. Oakbrook Terrace, IL: The Joint Commission.

Mangione, C. 2010. *Workforce training and preparedness*. Presentation at the Institute of Medicine workshop on Understanding What Works in Improving Health Literacy Within a State, November 30, 2010.

Marrone, L., S. Smith, M. J. Johnson, and E. Beck. 2010. *Independent study project*. San Diego, CA: UCSD.

NCIOM (North Carolina Institute of Medicine). 2007. *Just what did the doctor order?: Addressing low health literacy in North Carolina*. http://www.nciom.org/task-forces-and-projects/?task-force-on-health-literacy (accessed February 10, 2011).

NCIOM. 2010. *Just what did the doctor order?: Addressing low health literacy in North Carolina 2010 Update*. http://www.nciom.org/task-forces-and-projects/?task-force-on-health-literacy (accessed February 10, 2011).

Ratzan, S. C., and R. M. Parker. 2000. Introduction. In *National Library of Medicine current bibliographies in medicine: Health literacy*. NLM Pub. No. CBM 2000-1 ed., edited by C. Selden, M. Zorn, S. Ratzan, and R. Parker. Bethesda, MD: National Institutes of Health, U.S. Department of Health and Human Services.

Rudd, R. 2010. *Study circle guides*. Presentation at the Institute of Medicine workshop on Understanding What Works in Improving Health Literacy Within a State, November 30, 2010.

Saba, G. W., S. T. Wong, D. Schillinger, A. Fernandez, C. P. Sommkin, C. C. Wilson, and K. Grumback. 2006. Shared decision making and the experience of partnership in primary care. *Annals of Family Medicine* 4(1):54-62.

Sarkar, U., M. A. Handley, R. Gupta, A. Tang, E. Murphy, H. K. Seligman, K. G. Shojania, and D. Schillinger. 2008. Use of an interactive, telephone-based self-management support program to identify adverse events among ambulatory diabetes patients. *Journal of General Internal Medicine* 23(4):459-465.

Schillinger, D., M. Handley, F. Wang, and H. Hammer. 2009. Effects of self-management support on structure, process, and outcomes among vulnerable patients with diabetes: A three-arm practical clinical trial. *Diabetes Care* 32(4):559-566.

Schillinger, D. 2010. *The role of the university in improving health literacy.* Paper presented at the Institute of Medicine workshop on Understanding What Works in Improving Health Literacy Within a State, November 30, 2010.

Schwartzberg, J. G., A. Cowett, J. VanGeest, and M. S. Wolf. 2007. Communication techniques for patients with low health literacy: A survey of physicians, nurses, and pharmacists. *American Journal of Health Behavior* 31(Suppl 1):S96-S104.

Somers, S. A., and R. Mahadevan. 2010. *Health literacy implications of the Affordable Care Act.* Hamilton, NJ: Center for Health Care Strategies, Inc.

Sung, N. S., W. F. Crowley Jr., M. Genel, P. Salber, L. Sandy, L. M. Sherwood, S. B. Johnson, V. Catanese, H. Tilson, K. Getz, E. L. Larson, D. Scheinberg, E. A. Reece, H. Slavkin, A. Dobs, J. Grebb, R. A. Martinez, A. Korn, and D. Rimoin. 2003. Central challenges facing the national clinical research enterprise. *Journal of the American Medical Association* 289(10):1278-1287.

Turner, T., W. L. Cull, B. Bayldon, P. Klass, L. M. Sanders, M. P. Frintner, M. A. Abrams, and B. Dreyer. 2009. Pediatricians and health literacy: Descriptive results from a national survey. *Pediatrics* 124(Suppl):S299-S305.

Weiss, B. D., J. S. Blanchard, D. L. McGee, G. Hart, B. Warren, M. Burgoon, and K. J. Smith. 1994. Illiteracy among Medicaid recipients and its relationship to health care costs. *Journal of Health Care for the Poor and Underserved* 5(2):99-111.

Williams, M.V., R. M. Parker, D. W. Baker, N. S. Parikh, K. Pitkin, W. C. Coates, and J. R. Nurss. 1995. Inadequate functional health literacy among patients at two public hospitals. *Journal of the American Medical Association* 274(21):1677-1682.

Zimring, F. 1994. Carl Rogers. *Prospects: The quarterly review of comparative education.* 24(3/4):411-422. http://www.ibe.unesco.org/publications/ThinkersPdf/rogerse.PDF (accessed April 25, 2011).

Appendix A

Acronyms

AAMC	Association of American Medical Colleges
ACGME	Accreditation Council for Graduate Medical Education
ADAPT	Adaptation and Dissemination of AHRQ Comparative Effectiveness Research Products
AHEC	area health education center
AHRQ	Agency for Healthcare Research and Quality
AMA	American Medical Association
APHA	American Public Health Association
ATSM	automated telephone self-management
BMI	body mass index
CDC	Centers for Disease Control and Prevention
CHIP	Children's Health Insurance Program
CME	continuing medical education
CMS	Centers for Medicare and Medicaid Services
CTSI	Clinical and Translational Science Institute
ESL	English as a second language
FASHP	Federation of Associations of Schools of the Health Professions
GIS	geographic information system

HCI	Health Care Institute
HHS	Department of Health and Human Services
HIPAA	Health Insurance Portability and Accountability Act
HLI	Health Literacy Iowa
HLM	Health Literacy Missouri
HRSA	Health Resources and Services Administration
IHA	Institute for Healthcare Advancement
IOM	Institute of Medicine
LA	Los Angeles
LAC	Literacy Assistance Center
LCME	Liaison Committee on Medical Education
NAAL	National Assessment of Adult Literacy
NALS	National Adult Literacy Survey
NC	North Carolina
NCIOM	North Carolina Institute of Medicine
NCSALL	National Center for the Study of Adult Learning and Literacy
NIFL	National Institute For Literacy
NIH	National Institutes of Health
PHR	personal health records
PI	principal investigator
RA	rheumatoid arthritis
RDA	recommended daily allowance
SOPHE	Society for Public Health Educators
SRFCP	student-run free clinic program
UC	University of California
UCLA	University of California, Los Angeles
UCSD	University of California, San Diego
UCSF	University of California, San Francisco

Appendix B

Workshop Agenda

Understanding What Works in Health Literacy Across a State:
A Workshop

UCLA Sunset Village
Covel Commons
Grand Horizon Room

November 30, 2010

8:30–8:45	**Welcome and Introduction** *George Isham, M.D., M.S., Chair* *Institute of Medicine Roundtable on Health Literacy*
8:45–9:00	**Opening Remarks and Introduction of Keynote Speaker** *Alfred E. Osborne, Jr., Ph.D., M.B.A., M.A.* *Senior Associate Dean* *Anderson School of Management, UCLA*
9:00–9:20	**Keynote: Welcome and Overview of the Role of the University in Improving Health Literacy Statewide** *Eugene Washington, M.D., M.P.H.* *Vice Chancellor, UCLA Health Sciences* *Dean, David Geffen School of Medicine*
9:20–10:15	**State-Based Models to Improve Health Literacy**
9:20–9:40	The Road to Regional Transformation: The North Carolina Experience *Pam C. Silberman, Dr.P.H.* *President and CEO* *North Carolina Institute of Medicine*

9:20–9:40	The Iowa Experience: Creating a Shared Vision for Health Literacy in Iowa *Mary Ann Abrams, M.D., M.P.H.* *Center for Clinical Transformation* *Iowa Health System*
9:40–10:15	Discussion
10:15–10:40	**BREAK**
10:40–11:00	The Missouri Experience *Arthur Culbert, Ph.D.* *President and CEO* *Health Literacy Missouri*
11:00–11:20	Louisiana Statewide Health Initiative *Terry Davis, Ph.D.* *Professor* *Louisiana State University*
11:20–12:00	Discussion
12:00–1:00	**LUNCH**
1:00–2:30	**The Role of the University in Improving State Health Literacy**
1:00–1:20	How the University Can Advance State Health Literacy *Dean Schillinger, M.D.* *Professor of Clinical Medicine* *University of California, San Francisco*
1:20–1:40	Workforce Training and Preparedness. *Carol Mangione, M.D., M.S.P.H.* *Barbara A. Levey, M.D., & Gerald S. Levey, M.D.,* *Endowed Chair* *Professor of Medicine and Health Services* *University of California, Los Angeles*

1:40–2:00	How Health Literate Service Changes the Way in Which Things Are Done *Darren DeWalt, M.D., M.P.H.* (NOTE: Speaker was unable to attend the workshop so this subject was not covered.) *Associate Professor* *University of North Carolina at Chapel Hill*
2:00–2:30	Discussion
2:30–2:45	**BREAK**
2:45–4:30	**Improving Health Literacy at the Community Level**
2:45–3:05	New York City Mayor's Initiative on Health Literacy *Rima Rudd, M.S.P.H., Sc.D.* *Senior Lecturer on Society, Human Development, and Health* *Director of Education Programs* *Department of Society, Human Development, and Health* *Harvard School of Public Health*
3:05–3:20	MiVIA *Cynthia Solomon* *Chief Executive Officer* *FollowMe, Inc.*
3:20–3:40	Empowering Parents, Benefiting Children, Creating Strong Foundations for Health: Improving Health Literacy Through the Head Start Program *Ariella Herman, Ph.D., M.S.* *Research Director* *Health Care Institute* *Anderson School of Management* *University of California, Los Angeles*
3:40–4:00	Health Literacy at the UCSD Student-Run Free Clinic Project and Fellowship in Underserved Health Care *Ellen Beck, M.D.* *Director UCSD Student-Run Free Clinic Project and Fellowship in Underserved Health Care* *Director Medical Student Education and Clinical Professor, Department of Family and Preventive Medicine, UCSD School of Medicine*

4:00–4:30	Discussion
4:30–4:45	Recap of the Day's Discussion *George Isham*
5:00–7:00	**Reception and Presentation** **Covel Commons Terrace**
5:30	The Intersection of Public Health and Health Literacy *Jonathan Fielding, M.D., M.P.H.* *Director, Los Angeles County Department of Public Health* *County Health Officer, Los Angeles County*

Appendix C

Workshop Speaker Biosketches

Mary Ann Abrams, M.D., M.P.H., is in Clinical Performance Improvement at Iowa Health System (IHS), where she leads their health literacy efforts, and serves as faculty for Blank Children's Hospital Pediatric Residency Education Program in quality and community pediatrics. Dr. Abrams is co-chair of the American Academy of Pediatrics (AAP) Health Literacy Project Advisory Committee, and served on the AMA Health Literacy and Patient Safety Work Group. She is the Medical Director and Coalition Leader for Reach Out and Read (ROR)–Iowa. Dr. Abrams serves as the Iowa AAP Chapter's Community Access to Child Health (CATCH) Facilitator, and on the Iowa Medical Society Public Health Committee. She graduated from the University of Dayton, and received her medical degree from the Ohio State University College of Medicine, and her Master of Public Health from the Harvard University School of Public Health. She is board-certified in pediatrics and preventive medicine, and has extensive experience in both the clinical and public health arenas.

Ellen Beck, M.D., is Director of Community Education for the Division of Family Medicine of the Department of Family and Preventive Medicine at the University of California, San Diego (UCSD). She received her medical degree in 1976 from McGill University and completed a residency in family medicine. After serving as Director of the undergraduate program in Family Medicine at McGill University for two years, she joined the Department of Family and Preventive Medicine at UCSD as Predoctoral Director in 1988. With the help of UCSD medical students and several community partners, Dr. Beck co-founded three UCSD Student-Run Free Clinics in the San Diego community. These clinics provide free, quality medical, dental and social services to homeless and indigent people in Pacific Beach, Downtown and the Mountain View areas of San Diego. Her elective course "Community Advocacy" is one of the most popular courses offered to first year medical students through the School of Medicine. Dr. Beck also created a faculty development program, "Addressing the Health Needs of the Underserved," which is offered to physicians from all over the country. This program is designed to provide administrative, scholarly and teaching skills needed to develop and implement programs in primary care for the underserved. Sixty-six faculty members from 25 states have completed the program. In addition, she created a full-time 1 year Fellowship in Underserved Medicine at UCSD. She was appointed to the Healthy Families Advisory Panel in Sacramento, and is actively working on creating a collaborative Underserved Services Network for San Diego. Dr. Beck sees her work as "creating environments where individuals, families and communities take charge of their lives and achieve joy and wellbeing." Someday, she would like to have an impact on public education in this country, so that both schools and universities become centers that inspire creativity, wonder, a commitment to social justice, and a love of learning.

Arthur Culbert, Ph.D., is President and CEO of Health Literacy Missouri. Prior to being named President and CEO, Dr. Culbert served as Interim Executive Director of Health Literacy Missouri (HLM) and, since 2007, as the Senior Advisor to the Missouri Foundation for Health. In that role, he chaired the Missouri Health Literacy Enhancement Coordinating Council and facilitated the development of HLM, a statewide health literacy center. He has also been a leading force in building a national coalition of state health literacy initiatives and was recently selected to be a member of the Institute of Medicine's Roundtable on Health Literacy. Dr. Culbert spent 31 years as a faculty member and a dean at the Boston University schools of medicine and public health. He has more than 25 years of teaching experience in the fields of public health, medical sociology, and medical education. He has served as the National Chair for the Group on Student Affairs at the Association of American Medical Colleges. In the 1980s, he designed, developed and implemented the Early Medical School Selection Program. In the early 1990s, he authored Profile M.D., an electronic career advising program used by hundreds of medical students in medical schools throughout the country. Dr. Culbert writes a monthly guest column on health care for the *St. Louis Business Journal,* and has written several published articles regarding health literacy issues since 2007.

Terry C. Davis, Ph.D., is Professor of Medicine and Pediatrics at Louisiana State University Health Sciences Center in Shreveport, Louisian. For the past 25 years, she has led an interdisciplinary team investigating the impact of patient literacy on health and healthcare. Seminal achievements include development of the Rapid Estimate of Adult Literacy in Medicine, the most widely used literacy test in healthcare settings, and development of user-friendly patient education and provider training materials. Terry has authored more than 100 publications related to health literacy, health communication, and preventive medicine. She has served on Health Literacy Advisory Boards for both the American Medical Association and the American College of Physicians Foundation (ACP-F). Terry was an independent agent on the IOM Committee on Health Literacy and a developer of the AMA's Train-the-Trainer Health Literacy Curriculum. She is currently a member of the Healthy People 2010 Health Literacy/Health Communication Section and the FDA's Drug Safety and Risk Management Advisory Committee. Terry is the Principal Investigator (PI) on a 5-year NCI-funded grant to increase regular breast and CRC screening among patients with low literacy. She is also the PI on a national team that has developed and tested practical self-management diabetes and COPD guides and videos, which the ACP-F has distributed to more than a million patients. The team is working on a coronary artery disease guide. Currently, she is a co-investigator on a CDC-funded project to teach vaccine safety through the Academic Pediatric Association's online curriculum for residents and practicing physicians. Previously, she was a PI on several childhood immunization and newborn screening patient and provider education research projects funded by HRSA.

Darren A. DeWalt, M.D., M.P.H., is Assistant Professor in the Division of General Internal Medicine at the University of North Carolina (UNC) at Chapel Hill School of Medicine. Dr. DeWalt actively researches self-management interventions for patients with low literacy and focuses on chronic diseases like diabetes, heart failure, and asthma. His focus is on patient-physician communication and health system design to achieve better outcomes for vulnerable populations. He is the principal investigator at the UNC research site for the Patient Reported Outcomes Measurement Information System (PROMIS) and chair of the Pediatrics Workgroup. Dr. DeWalt is a former Robert Wood Johnson Clinical Scholar at UNC. He completed his residency in internal medicine and pediatrics at UNC where he also served as chief resident in internal medicine. He received his medical degree from the Vanderbilt University School of Medicine. Dr. DeWalt led the design team and is currently a national improvement advisor for the Improving Performance in Practice (IPIP) program for the boards and specialty societies of internal medicine, family medicine, and pediatrics.

Jonathan Fielding, M.D., M.P.H., M.A., M.B.A., is a Professor of Health Services and Pediatrics and Co-Director of the UCLA Center for Healthier Children, Families and Communities. Dr. Fielding serves as Director of Public Health and Health Officer for Los Angeles County where he is responsible for the full range of public health activities for 10 million county residents. Dr. Fielding teaches Determinants of Health and participates as faculty lecturer in several of the Department courses. He received both his M.D., M.A. (History of Science), and M.P.H. from Harvard University, and his M.B.A. from the Wharton School of Business Administration. His areas of expertise include the development of clinical preventive services guidelines, prevention economics and financing, and health promotion for children, adults and families in community, clinical and occupational settings. As the founding Co-Director of the Center for Health Enhancement, Education and Research, he provided the first comprehensive university-based center to focus on clinical and worksite prevention opportunities. He formerly served as the Founding Board Member, Chairman of the Board and member of the Executive Committee of The California Wellness Foundation, the largest U.S. Foundation devoted to disease prevention and health promotion, and is among the 50 largest U.S. Foundations. Further, he was a founding member of the U.S. Preventive Services Task Force and is Vice-Chair, Community Preventive Services Task Force. He is immediate past President of the American College of Preventive Medicine. Dr. Fielding's awards include the Porter Prize, given for his national impact on improving the lives of Americans; and membership in the National Academy of Sciences' Institute of Medicine. He is the author of more than 150 original scientific articles and chapters, Editor of *Annual Review of Public Health*, and Associate Editor of the textbook *Public Health and Preventive Medicine*.

Ariella Herman, Ph.D., is a Senior Lecturer of Operations and Decision Sciences at the UCLA Anderson School of Management. She is the Research Director of the Johnson & Johnson Head Start Programs and is the founder of the UCLA/Johnson & Johnson Health Care Institute. Prior to joining the UCLA faculty, Dr. Herman was a tenured Associate Professor in the Management Science Department at the Ecole Superieur de Commerce de Paris (ESCP), France. Her research and consulting have been in the areas of child care and health care management systems. In the last 10 years her main focus has been on low income population and developing low literacy health education programs. Through the Health Care Institute, her research has shown that the healthcare system could save millions of dollars annually in direct costs associated with unnecessary emergency room and doctor/clinic visits. She is a key contributor to several programs conducted by the Harold and Pauline Price Center for Entrepreneurial Studies at UCLA Anderson and serves as an instructor in the Head Start-Johnson & Johnson Management Fellows Program, as well as several UCLA Anderson Executive Education courses. Ms. Herman has received several awards for outstanding teaching, including the Citibank teaching award in 1995. She was recognized with the Head Start-Johnson & Johnson Exceptional Teaching Award and the Health Literacy Award for the "most innovative health education and promotion rogram" in 2009. Most recently, Dr. Herman was awarded the first annual Health Literacy Innovation Champions Award by Health Literacy Innovations, for her work in the Health Care Institute. Dr. Herman, who is fluent in Hebrew, French, Italian, Romanian, German, Spanish, and English, earned her undergraduate degree in mathematics from the University of Paris, a master's in engineering from UCLA, and a Ph.D. in management from the University of Paris. Most recently, her research with the Health Care Institute has been published in the *Journal of Community Health*, *Journal of Emergency Medicine*, and has been featured in several high-profile news publications.

George Isham, M.D., M.S., is Medical Director and Chief Health Officer for HealthPartners. He is responsible for quality and utilization management, chairs the Benefits Committee, and leads Partners for Better Health, a program and strategy for improving member health. Before his current position, Dr. Isham was medical director of MedCenters Health Plan in Minneapolis. In the late 1980s, he was executive director of University Health Care, an organization affiliated with the University of Wisconsin, Madison. Dr. Isham received his Master of Science in preventive medicine/administrative medicine at the University of Wisconsin, Madison, and his Doctor of Medicine from the University of Illinois. He completed an internship and residency in internal medicine at the University of Wisconsin Hospital and Clinics in Madison. His experience as a primary care physician included 8 years at the Freeport Clinic in Freeport, Illinois, and 3 years as clinical assistant professor in medicine at the University of Wisconsin. HealthPartners is a consumer-governed Minnesota health plan that formed through the 1992 affiliation of Group Health, Inc., and MedCenters Health Plan. HealthPartners is a large managed health care organization in Minnesota, representing nearly 800,000 members. Group Health, founded in 1957, is a network of staff medical and dental centers located throughout the Twin Cities. MedCenters, founded in 1972, is a network of contracted physicians serving members through affiliated medical and dental centers.

Carol M. Mangione, M.D., M.S.P.H., is the Barbara A. Levey, M.D. & Gerald S. Levey, M.D. Endowed Chair and Professor of Medicine and Health Services at UCLA. Dr. Mangione is the Director of the NIH/ NIA funded UCLA/Drew Resource Center for Minority Aging Research/ Center for Health Improvement of Minority Elderly (RCMAR III/ CHIME II), and Co-director of the UCLA Robert Wood Johnson Clinical Scholars Program. In both of these programs she mentors and trains physicians developing research careers. Dr. Mangione is the principal investigator for the Translational Research Centers for Diabetes Within Managed-Care Settings (TRIAD) Legacy study, funded by the Centers for Disease Control and Prevention (CDC) and the National Institute of Diabetes and Digestive and Kidney Diseases (NIDDK) to study the quality of care for persons with diabetes where her work has focused on the relationship between organization of care, cost sharing, control of cardiovascular risk factors and process outcomes such as adherence to medications. She was also recently awarded funding from CDC and NIDDK to conduct the "Diabetes Health Plan: A System Level Intervention to Prevent and Treat Diabetes," and was appointed to be the National Chairperson for the multi-site National Program entitled "Natural Experiments and Effectiveness Studies for Diabetes Prevention and Control." Dr. Mangione is also principal investigator of the Agency for Healthcare Research and Quality (AHRQ) Virtual Lab for California Project. The purpose of this project is to create a coalition of government, academic, and private entities within the state of California to provide access to a diverse set of existing data to answer research questions relating to the health of women and minorities across the life span. Currently, Dr. Mangione serves as co-investigator of the National Heart Lung and Blood Institute funded project entitled Comparative Effectiveness and Outcomes Improvement (CEOI). This project is a statewide effort that aims to develop sustainable statewide infrastructure for Comparative Effectiveness Research on primary and secondary prevention of cardiovascular disease among managed care populations. Dr. Mangione received her B.S. from the University of Michigan, Ann Arbor, her M.D. degree from the University of California, San Francisco, and her M.S.P.H. from the Harvard School of Public Health, Boston.

Alfred E. Osborne, Jr., Ph.D., M.B.A., M.A., is Senior Associate Dean of UCLA Anderson. In this role, he oversees a variety of key areas and initiatives within the school, including development, alumni relations, career and corporate initiatives, career management, marketing and communications and executive education. Dr. Osborne is also professor of Global Economics & Management and founder and faculty director of the Harold Price Center for Entrepreneurial Studies at UCLA. The Price Center serves to organize all faculty research and student activities and curricula related to the study of entrepreneurship and new business development at UCLA Anderson. A corporate governance expert, Dr. Osborne formed a Director Education and Certification Program designed to help officers and directors of private firms prepare for the higher level of scrutiny that comes when they take their companies public. This program also educates directors and officers regarding SEC regulations, FASB considerations, NASDAQ rules and the current best practices in corporate governance. Dr. Osborne currently serves as a director of Kaiser Aluminum and the Heckmann Corporation, and has served many years on the corporate boards of Times Mirror Company, US Filter Corporation, Greyhound Lines, Inc., First Interstate Bank of California, Nordstrom, Inc. and K2, Inc., among others. He has served as an economic fellow at the Brookings Institution and directed studies at the SEC that contributed to changes in Rule 144, Regulation D, and other exemptive requirements to the securities laws designed to lower costs and improve liquidity and capital market access to venture capitalists and emerging growth firms alike. Dr. Osborne's current research interests include venture capital and private equity, and the role of the board of directors in private and public corporations. He remains active in the entrepreneurial and venture development community, has served on the editorial boards of several journals, and consults with growing companies and nonprofit organizations on business and economic matters.

Rima Rudd, Sc.D., M.S.P.H., is Senior Lecturer on Society, Human Development, and Health at the Harvard School of Public Health. Her work centers on health communication and the design and evaluation of public health programs. She teaches courses on innovative strategies in health education, program planning and evaluation, health literacy, and theory. Dr. Rudd is focusing her research inquiries on literacy related disparities and literacy related barriers to health programs, services, and care. She works closely with the adult education, public health, oral health, and medical sectors and with several national literacy initiatives in Canada, England, and Europe. Dr. Rudd wrote several reports that are helping shape the agenda in health literacy research and practice. They include the health literacy chapter of the Health and Human Services book *Communicating Health: Priorities and Strategies for Progress* (2003) and the Educational Testing Services report, *Literacy and Health in America* (2004). She introduced the concept of a "health literacy environment" that is shaping examinations of barriers to care in hospitals, health centers, and social service agencies. Her long-standing emphasis on the dual components of literacy: social system demands and the skills of individuals has reshaped definition of terms with a focus on health literacy as an interaction and not simply a characteristic of individuals. She served on the Institute of Medicine Committee on Health Literacy, on the National Research Council Committee on Measuring Adult Literacy, on the Joint Commission Advisory Committee on Health Literacy and Patient Safety. She currently serves on several national advisory boards and is principal investigator and co-principal investigator on several health literacy research inquiries. Dr. Rudd serves as Senior Health Literacy Advisor to the Missouri Foundation and holds appointments as Visiting Professor at London South Bank University and as Visiting Senior Scholar at the Horowitz Health Literacy Center, University of Maryland School of Public Health. Rima Rudd is considered a leader in this new field of inquiry.

Dean Schillinger, M.D., is a practicing primary care physician at San Francisco General Hospital (SFGH), an urban public hospital, where he sees patients, teaches in the primary care residency program, and conducts research as a member of the UCSF Primary Care Research Center. In his administrative capacities, he has directed the Medi-Cal managed care clinic at SFGH, the ambulatory care clinics at SFGH, and has been the Director of Clinical Operations for the Department of Medicine. He is currently the Director of the UCSF Center for Vulnerable Populations, a new research center committed to transforming clinical and public health practice and policy to improve health and health care for socially vulnerable people. Dr. Schillinger has focused his research on health care for vulnerable populations, including the impact of managed care, improving systems of care for publicly insured and uninsured patients, and most recently, health communication. His current work has focused on literacy, health communication, and chronic disease prevention and management. He has carried out a number of studies exploring the impact of limited health literacy on the care of patients with diabetes and heart disease, and was honored with the 2003 Institute for Healthcare Advancement Research Award for this work. He was recently awarded grants from the National Institutes of Health, The California Endowment, the Commonwealth Fund, the Agency for Healthcare Research and Quality, and the California Health Care Foundation, to develop and evaluate disease-management programs tailored to the literacy and language needs of patients with chronic disease, and is a co-investigator for the National Association of Public Health and Hospital Institute's Diabetes Quality Improvement Consortium. Dr. Schillinger contributed to the 2004 Institute of Medicine Report on Health Literacy, is a section editor for the textbooks *Understanding Health Literacy* (AMA press) and *Caring for Vulnerable and Underserved Populations* (Lange series, 2007), and is a former member of the American College of Physician's Health Communication Advisory Board. He completed an Open Society Institute Advocacy Fellowship working with California Literacy, Inc., a nonprofit educational organization that helps people gain literacy skills, to advance the California Health Literacy Initiative. He recently returned from a semester as Visiting Scholar at the University of Chile School of Public Health to help develop chronic disease prevention and treatment initiatives.

Pam C. Silberman, J.D., Dr.Ph., is the President and CEO of the North Carolina Institute of Medicine (NCIOM). In the last year, she has helped to staff task forces on Prevention, Access to Care, Adolescent Health, Behavioral Health Needs of the Military and their Families, Co-Location of Different Populations in Adult Care Homes, and work to develop Healthy North Carolina 2020 goals and objectives. In recent years, she has also helped staff task forces on Substance Abuse Services, and Transitions for People with Intellectual or Other Developmental Disabilities, Health Literacy, Primary Care and Specialty Supply, Chronic Kidney Disease, the Ethical Issues that would Arise in Event of an Influenza Pandemic, Covering the Uninsured, the Health Care Safety Net, Nursing Workforce, Latino Health, NC Health Choice, Long-Term Care, and Dental Care Access. Dr. Silberman is also the Publisher of the *North Carolina Medical Journal*. She serves as Associate Director for Policy Analysis with the Cecil G. Sheps Center for Health Services Research at UNC. She is a Clinical Associate Professor in the Department of Health Policy and Management, Gillings School of Global Public Health at UNC, and teaches courses on underserved populations and safety-net programs. Dr. Silberman served on numerous legislative Commissions, including NC Legislative Study Commission on Medicaid Reform (2003–2005), Managed Care (2000–2001), Access to Health Insurance (1991–1993); and Indigent Care (1985–1989).

Cynthia Solomon is a nationally recognized Health Advocate and the Founder and President, of FollowMe, Inc. a Personal Health Record company launched in 2000. Her organization specializes in developing customized Personal Health Records for vulnerable populations such as www.mivia.org, a PHR initially developed for migrant and seasonal farm workers launched in 2003 and www.healthshack.info, a PHR developed for Homeless and System Based Youth launched January 2010 as well as www.followmyheart.org, a PHR developed in partnership with Children's National Medical Center and the American College of Cardiology for patients diagnosed with congenital heart disease launched October 2010. Ms. Solomon participated as a member of the Markle Foundation *Connecting for Health* Workgroup in developing the recommendations and standards for interoperability between electronic health records (EHRs) and personal health records (PHRs). She has presented testimony on PHR technology to the NCVHS NHII workgroup and the Consumer Empowerment Workgroup–American Health Information Community on the role of Government in PHR technology and the Presidential IT Commission on Interoperability (www.endingthedocumentgame.gov), as well as the IOM Roundtable on Health Literacy and the ONC HIT Policy Committee, Using HIT to Eliminate Disparities. She is currently serving on the ONC Health IT Workgroup and Panel "Understanding the Impact of Health IT in Underserved Communities."

A. Eugene Washington, M.D., M.Sc., assumed his role as Vice Chancellor and Dean in February 2010. He is an internationally renowned clinical investigator and health-policy scholar whose wide-ranging research has been instrumental in shaping national health policy and practice guidelines. As Vice Chancellor and Dean, Dr. Washington oversees the UCLA Health System and the David Geffen School of Medicine, and serves as the principal spokesperson for health sciences at UCLA. Prior to coming to UCLA, Dr. Washington served as Executive Vice Chancellor and Provost for UCSF, where he co-founded the Medical Effectiveness Research Center for Diverse Populations. He also co-founded the UCSF-Stanford Evidence-based Practice Center and, from 1996 to 2004, chaired the Department of Obstetrics, Gynecology, and Reproductive Sciences. He has published extensively in his major areas of research, which include prenatal genetic testing, cervical cancer screening and prevention, non-cancerous uterine conditions management, reproductive tract infections, quality of healthcare and racial/ethnic disparities in health outcomes. Dr. Washington has earned numerous honors and awards, including the Outstanding Service Medal from the U.S. Public Health Service, and election to the IOM of the National Academy of Sciences, where he serves on the governing Council of IOM. He also serves on the boards of the Robert Wood Johnton Foundation, the California Wellness Foundation, and the congressionally mandated Scientific Management Review Board of the National Institutes of Health.